Multiple Sclerosis...
Why _Not_ Me?

by

Vincent Spoto

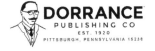

DORRANCE
PUBLISHING CO
EST. 1920
PITTSBURGH, PENNSYLVANIA 15238

Dorrance Publishing Co
585 Alpha Drive
Suite 103
Pittsburgh, PA 15238
Visit our website at *www.dorrancebookstore.com*

ISBN: 978-1-4809-3062-9
eISBN: 978-1-4809-3039-1

Contents

To my wife Luisa,
and my children,
Deanna and Lauren – Thank you!

Preface

Multiple Sclerosis...Why Not Me? is the non-fiction account of the author, Vincent Spoto, and his struggles with Multiple Sclerosis (MS). After his diagnosis and in the beginning stages of the disease, Vincent often wondered "why me?" and did not think it was fair that he was amongst the chosen individuals destined to endure the journey called MS. After Vincent's MS became more advanced, he had to use a cane to walk and had a hard time functioning as he once did. This is when he began to open-up and talk with others who may have been wondering, when thinking about his plight, "why me?" themselves. Vincent has decided to use his disease for the greater good, and has written this manuscript in an attempt to appeal to readers who are in similar situations and are looking for someone with whom they can relate. His story also serves as an inspiration to others dealing with their own medical challenges aside from MS. The many examples he provides of how he has made adjustments to a host of daily routines in order to continue supporting an active lifestyle, all while maintaining a positive attitude and keeping an optimistic outlook for the future, will hopefully encourage others to do the same.

Individuals wishing to learn more about Vincent's journey with MS can contact him via email at *vincentspoto1@gmail.com.*

Acknowledgments

My inspirations for writing this book are many, and I am certain I may have omitted the names of a few people who have helped encourage me along the way. So please, forgive me. I'm sure that after reading this, those whom I may have neglected to mention will know who they are, so please accept my apologies in advance, as it is difficult remembering to mention everyone. But, here goes...

First, I'd like to acknowledge my personal trainer, Christopher Mills. In 2011, I decided to utilize the services of a personal trainer, and that's when I met Chris. Prior to that (and several times thereafter), I tried various physical therapy routines, but rarely felt challenged. Chris pushes me just far enough; he inspires me to stay active by alternating my bi-weekly training sessions that I have with him, doing balance and core/upper body strength workouts, respectively. Chris gives me the confidence and motivation I need to keep moving. I usually go to the gym once or twice per week on my own, plus I see Chris on two other days of the week. That's three to four days per week of active exercise! This is something that gets me out there, keeps me moving and helps me cope with my MS. Chris always mentions to me that he wishes he had started working with me a few years sooner right after my diagnosis so that perhaps he could have positively impacted my impaired mobility.

I wish the same. But, I'm thankful at this time that I have Chris to help inspire me, build my confidence and keep my body in shape and ready for when the "cure" happens! Thank you, Chris!

I'd also next like to thank my next-door neighbors, Leslie and Jerry Roschwalb. Leslie and Jerry are always there for me and willing to help out my wife Luisa, our children and me with even the most trivial things. They also lend much needed strength and emotional support to Lusia, who silently deals each and every day with my having MS. The nice thing about Leslie and Jerry is that they never treat me any differently because I have MS and will not coddle or pamper me/give me special treatment when we're out (unless I'm having a difficult time and ask for help). Thanks guys, for always being there to listen, help out and lend support!

Next, my business partners Allen Gutterman and Brian Lin continue to support me. Since we started RRMS Advisors in 2008 (my consulting and advisory business), both Allen and Brian have always encouraged me every step of the way. I occupy shared office space with them in Manhattan, and usually commute from Long Island into New York City three to four days per week. Whenever we go out on sales calls or visit with prospective clients to do marketing pitches, I am grateful for their patience and always very thankful for the way in which they help me navigate my way around various cities, office buildings, airports, hotels, restaurants, etc. As Allen always says whenever I thank him, "Don't be silly, there's no need to thank me. You're my friend." Despite what he says, I want to send a special thank you to both Allen and Brian for putting up with me and for always helping me out!

Special thanks to Brian Bluver, who is Chief Legal Counsel for my business. I often look to Brian to proof my work. Throughout writing this book, I placed a great deal of reliance on Brian's proofreading and editing skills. No matter how busy he was, Brian would always find time to assist. I am grateful for the time he has spent helping me with this manuscript and reviewing drafts of each chapter to see if they were logical, easy to read and made sense. I appreciate the suggestions, inputs and edits Brian has offered, particularly relating to the help he's provided relating to suggesting names for certain chapter titles. Thank you, Brian!

I would also like to thank Dr. Karen Blitz-Shabbir, the neurologist whose care I have been under since I was diagnosed with MS in 2006. Between regular check-ups, steroid infusions and refill maintenance to my Baclofen pump, I see Dr. Blitz on average about six times per year. And each time I see her, I always begin my visits with the same question: "Has a cure been found yet?" Lately, Dr. Blitz pre-empts me from asking the question and, before I can even greet her to say hello, she starts off each visit by saying, "No cure yet, but they're working on it." Since I have started seeing Dr. Blitz, I have followed her recommendations and have changed treatment options a number of times. She continues to monitor my condition and will occasionally suggest new and alternative treatments, reminding me that MS affects everyone differently and while therapies available to date are designed to slow or stop progression of the disease, one can never tell what effect a specific therapy may have on a person. I admire Dr. Blitz's aggressive nature, and the fact that she seldom waits for me to ask my famous "cure" question. Thank you, Dr. Blitz, for putting up with me and for helping me through this difficult journey!

To my late father-in-law Mario Conte, who passed away in 1998, long before I was diagnosed with MS. Ever since I met him, I always viewed Mr. Conte as a special man. He was nothing other than kind and helpful to me, my parents, Luisa, Deanna and Lauren. Born in Italy and held as a prisoner of war by the Nazis while serving in the Italian army during WWII, Mr. Conte was a strong, courageous and respectful man who left this earth way too soon. He never spoke of his prisoner of war days, as I'm sure they were horrible and he did not care to burden others with his stories. I would be remiss without mentioning him and expressing my deep gratitude for all he has done for me and my family! I know if he were alive today, he'd be inundating me with MS research summaries and news about clinical trials, experimental drugs, pioneering neurologists at the top of their field and Complementary and Alternative Medicine (CAM) suggestions. He was truly very special. I miss you, Dad! Words cannot express my special thanks for all your help. I know you are looking down from heaven and continuing to watch over me!

Special thanks too to my mother-in-law Angelina Conte, who to this day at the age of 88 provides our family with her endless love and support. She's been living by herself in the same house in Howard Beach, Queens since my father-in-law's passing in 1998. God bless her, as she remains strong and independent. Up until recently, she had to be reminded each September not to climb on a ladder to pick fruit from the fig trees that are planted in her backyard, and is always offering to cook something to eat. What a strong and courageous woman she is, and what an inspiration she continues to be. Thanks, Mom, for your love and support!

To my children, Deanna and Lauren. I am proud of both of you and thank you for being there and for helping support me and your mom along my journey. I know it's not easy for either of you knowing your dad has this thing called MS, and I truly appreciate your support and love. If there is any consolation in my having MS, it has to be that it did not afflict me until after you were both in your late teens and not as youngsters growing-up. I'm so thankful that I was able to play with both of you, visit amusement parks with both of you, take cruises with both of you, go to ballgames with both of you, and yes—do the Disney thing with both of you! My only request is that you turn off the lights in your rooms when leaving and that you continue to be there for one another! Thank you, Deanna and Lauren, for your help, support and love, and for giving me a reason to stay active by going into your rooms after you leave them to shut-off the lights!

A special and heartfelt thanks goes out to my wife Luisa for putting up with me since we got married in 1984 (and a few years prior to that too!), and for helping and supporting me throughout my journey. When you think of MS, you often think of the person who has the disease and the stress, physical and emotional toll it takes on *them*. But, seldom does one think of the emotional toll and stress MS takes on the spouse and caregiver. Luisa, I know I may not always acknowledge it, but I am truly grateful and thankful for your caring, admire your strength and appreciate the love and support that you provide. If I seem aloof at times and let things roll off my shoulders, make strange faces when I'm feeling frustrated or "snap back" for no reason, I hope you will understand why. As for not appearing to be bothered and letting things pass, MS has certainly taught me to shrug off the "little things" and soften my approach to dealing with many things in life. I am thankful for all that you have done and continue to do for me, Deanna and Lauren. Thank you, "Weezie!"

And lastly, it goes without saying that I owe everything to my parents, Rosalie and Joseph Spoto.

My mom, Rosalie Spoto, passed away in 2009 at the age of 84 and never knew I had MS. She did, however surmise that something was amiss. For example, a year or so *before* I was officially diagnosed in 2006 when I had no reason to even see a doctor, my mom would repeatedly ask me why I was limping. This was something I swear to this day that I was not doing. Clearly, though, she saw something that was not quite right. My mom was always very proud of me and would frequently "embarrass" me in front of others by bragging about my accomplishments. I remember back in 1989 when I was working for Citibank and was promoted to Vice President, she would tell everyone she saw in the years that followed that *"My son, Vincent, is* the *Vice President of*

Citibank!" She constantly boasted about my brothers and I, our wives, her grandchildren and my dad's heroic wartime adventures. For example, she would repeatedly tell everyone she met (i.e. store owners, doctors, nurses, complete strangers, etc.) that her husband Joe made sixty-nine parachute jumps during WWII, was wounded in action, received a purple heart and was a member of General MacArthur's Honor Guard, etc. Our unassuming homes were consistently portrayed to others by my mom as "Beverly Hills mansions," and the modest cars we drove described to others as if they were "Rolls Royces."

My mom was also a very generous and caring person. Whenever she won a small prize at bingo or would get lucky *more than* once in a while with a scratch-off lottery ticket or from playing a daily lottery number (she had this uncanny sense about picking and playing winning numbers she dreamt about the night before), she would be quick to send each of her three sons a small check with a portion of her winnings. I loved when she played and "hit" on a lottery number or won at bingo, as that usually resulted in extra cash in my pocket. I know if she were alive today, she'd be proud of the way I'm managing my MS (and of course, would be very concerned and supportive nonetheless), and call me each day with a reminder to take my medications and to be sure and rest. And she'd probably say: "See, I knew something was wrong, as I always said you were limping." I miss you mom, and want to thank you for a lifetime of support and for continuing to look over me!

My dad, Joseph, who passed in 2014 at the age of ninety-one as I was midway through writing this book, was a purple-heart veteran paratrooper of the Second World War. He came to this country from Italy at age six not speaking any English, and grew up in the great depression. By far, along with my late father-in law Mario Conte, the two of them were amongst the strongest men I have ever known. My father would endlessly recount stories from WWII, always remembering the most intimate details. Things like: (i) how he made sixty-nine parachute jumps during the war, or (ii) how he was awarded the purple heart after saving members of his battalion in the Philippines who fell under enemy attack, or (iii) after being wounded, how he then had to be evacuated for treatment from the combat zone strapped to the wing of a small sea plane, or (iv) how he avoided enemy fire by crawling along the ground and taking cover in ditches, or (v) how he was brought to the basement of a church by the Philippine people and pretended to be dead as he was hidden in an empty casket to avoid being captured by the Japanese, or (vi) about how he was selected to be a member of General MacArthur's Honor Guard and was signaled out to sail home from the South Pacific with the Marines on the USS Intrepid when the war ended in 1945.

And this is just the tip of the iceberg regarding his wartime stories!

Each of his stories reminds me of just what a strong and courageous man he really was. I often think of how difficult his life must have been coming to this country at age six as Italian immigrant, growing up in the Great Depression, fighting in the South Pacific jungles during World War II, raising three children with my mom in a small and very modest five room house which had only one telephone, one bathroom and one black-and-white television set (without a remote control, I might add), holding down a modest white color job bringing home only simple wages and living alone after my mom passed for nearly five years in the same house that my brothers and I were raised in.

And I cannot forget the fact that growing up, my dad would spend countless hours all throughout my grammar and junior high school years helping me study for spelling tests, prepare projects for upcoming school science fairs, help me write essays and compose stories, etc. He did this no matter how tired and under the weather he was feeling after a long, hard day at work. I am blessed to have pretty decent organizational and writing skills (I think), and owe my strengths and abilities here to my dad. He was a strong supporter of education, and made schooling for my brothers and me a top priority. And, he never missed a "meet the teacher" or "open school night" either! He would always tell me to "do the best you can" and worried less about the grades my brothers and I got and more about the effort we put into studying and preparing for exams. God help us if we failed an exam that we did not put in a 100-percent effort studying for!

This gives me pause to think back and reflect on my disability and the many challenges that having MS creates. By far, my dad, my mom, my mother-in-law and my father-in-law had it a lot more difficult than do I, and I consider myself fortunate to be able to draw upon their strengths and courage to continue on.

I want you to know dad that I am going to beat this MS thing, rest assured. And do me a favor, please let mom and Mr. Conte know that too! Thanks for everything, dad!

Introduction and Foreword

When I was first diagnosed with Multiple Sclerosis (MS) at the age of forty-seven in the summer of 2006, I would frequently ask myself, "Why me?"

During the early stages of this disease, my symptoms were virtually invisible. At first, the annoyance of having to take a weekly injection and the reality that I could no longer withstand the summertime heat, worship the sun and go to the beach as I once did were my only real issues. At the point during which I was first diagnosed, Multiple Sclerosis was just a name. I think Annette Funicello had something called MS (but I never really followed her life), so I had no idea what its impact was. Then, there is Montel Williams, the television personality and talk show host; he looks normal...and Neil Cavuto, the anchor on Fox News, he looks normal too. And oh yeah, I can't forget Squiggy from the 1970s television show *Laverne & Shirley*. He appeared to be normal too (I think)! I do remember Richard Pryor having MS, though, and the debilitating affect which the disease, combined with his hard lifestyle, had on him. Each one of these figures has been afflicted with MS somewhat differently, and I know that both Richard Pryor and Annette Funicello have since passed away (although I understand not directly from MS itself). So, how bad could this MS thing really be?

Then, I did some further research on the internet. After a bunch of Google searches and a fair amount of reading and investigation, I thought: Oh my God, this thing called MS is *not* good! Not good at all!

As time went on and my walking, fatigue, balance and tolerance to heat became more of a challenge, I would constantly ask myself the "Why me?" question. As I came to slowly accept my condition and began to look around, I started to realize that there were much worse things in life to have, and that almost everyone had their own individual problems and crosses to bear. I don't want to kid anyone though; it took me over five years to get to this point. Even today, I'm not sure I am fully there yet. There are still days when the "Why me?" question resonates throughout my brain, and it takes some time before I compose myself, reflect a bit and think, "Why *not* me?" And on these days, I still do sometimes feel down and depressed.

Granted, having MS is not something I would wish on anyone. I truly wish I did not have it. But clearly, there are worse things in life to deal with. Rather than constantly deny I have MS, I now consider myself somewhat fortunate that a worse fate has not been dealt to me. Don't get me wrong—having MS sucks. It *really* sucks! <u>*REALLY SUCKS!!!*</u> So, feeling down and depressed does occur on occasion, but I try to bounce-back and not let these feelings take-over. The frustration however, is not just something I feel occasionally; instead, it is something that I live with almost daily.

But like some others, I am not going to pretend and say things like "MS is the best thing that has ever happened to me," or "being diagnosed with MS has been a blessing in disguise," or "having MS has taught me many lessons in life." No, having MS does suck! But, I am a realist and constantly remind myself that "it could be a lot worse."

Funny, when I was first diagnosed with MS in 2006, I had no reason or the slightest desire to share my diagnosis with anyone. In fact, I made a conscious effort *not* to disclose it. At first, only my wife Luisa was aware. Shortly thereafter, we shared the news with our daughters Deanna and Lauren. As life went on over the next few years, I told no one else: Not my parents, not my brothers, not my mother-in-law, not any other relatives, not my employer, not my work colleagues, not my close friends, not my neighbors, not my business partners—no one. Like I said, my symptoms were virtually invisible (except to my mom), so there was no reason to share anything. I kept my feelings to myself of what the future may hold, and did not say a word to anyone. Since there were truly no symptoms at first, I really had no frustrations. I did not really have any significant limitations and therefore had nothing really to complain about.

In 2009, a few years after my initial diagnosis, I developed a slight limp and there were infrequent and isolated occasions where business colleagues and friends would ask, "Why are you limping?" My reaction would be to shrug it off, deny I was limping or respond by saying that I had injured my knee or had purchased a new pair of shoes that were hurting my feet and needed to be broken in. For the most part people bought it (I think), and I moved on. I'm sure others who may have noticed did not ask or say anything. Those that I told may have silently wondered if something more serious was wrong and disbelieved me. Only my mom, who passed away in November 2009, was relentless in her querying and would _not_ accept my denials that nothing was wrong or that I had hurt my knee. In fact, my mom would ask me even one year or so before I was formally diagnosed in 2006: "Why are you limping?" I swear I had no visible signs of impairment (or so I thought) and didn't even know that I had MS, let alone did I understand what it was. Leave it to a mother though, to know when something is amiss with their child!

Toward the end of 2010 and in early 2011, my limp became more outwardly visible and my balance was becoming an issue. So, I gave in and began to utilize a cane to help me walk better and keep my balance.

It was at this point in time that I needed to "open my closet doors" and level with relatives, colleagues, close friends and neighbors. It was time to tell people the truth. Be open. Be honest. The fact that I had an issue had now become more visible, and I could not hide things any longer; I guess the cane was a dead give-away. MS was no longer an invisible thing! By now, however, my mom had passed away. So, I couldn't tell her.

At first, having MS was a very difficult thing for me to share. I remember first telling my two brothers, and next my dad. My eyes teared-up and the stress associated with this disclosure was unnerving. I remember telling people at first that I had a mild case of MS (I'm not sure that such a thing even existed), and that I was fine. I next opened up to my business partners, selected work colleagues and relatives, close neighbors and a few intimate friends. Each time, I had to hold-back the eye tearing and overcome the crackling in my voice. However, everyone I did tell was very supportive and accepting, and many asked, "What is MS?" It was not easy for me, especially since I was not really certain myself of what exactly it was. And even today, there are times when disclosing it to others is not always easy.

I keep my explanation about what MS is very short and simple, using the analogy of a wire that has become frayed or has tattered insulation. I generally say something like: "Picture the wires that connect your brain to different parts of your body and carry signals to them. Well, MS is what's referred to as an autoimmune disease in which the good cells that fight and ward-off the bad disease guys mistakenly take the insulation which covers the wires, called myelin, as a bad guy. In MS, the immune system gets confused and attacks the myelin and nerves leading to the brain and spinal cord. So, the good cells start to munch away and destroy. Soon, the underlying wires become exposed and the protective insulation, the myelin, becomes frayed or destroyed. In some cases, the actual wires themselves, or axons, become severed or damaged. As such, signals that are sent from the brain to various parts of the body are transmitted more slowly or indirectly, or are not transmitted completely at all.

Everyone that has MS is impacted differently; in my case, the wires that are damaged go to my left leg, and impair my strength and balance. (Thank goodness it is not my right leg, and I am still able to drive)! My brain says: 'Okay, left leg, it's time to lift and walk.' But my left leg does not get the full message, may get it more slowly or does not get it at all. (Now I know how my wife Luisa feels every time she asks me to do something and the message just goes into one ear and out the other). So today I limp, have some trouble walking, get fatigued more easily and have difficulty at times maintaining my balance. Luckily though, I have only experienced one or two falls since my diagnosis.

This explanation that I use to describe this horrible disease to others has become standard. Clearly, it is not something out of the Harvard Medical School dictionary, but it is nonetheless a description that is concise, simplistic and easy for everyone to understand. Even I understand it when I tell others! There is no need to get into the fact that roughly eighty-five percent of MS patients are initially diagnosed with the relapsing-remitting form of the disease, and that about fifty percent of these individuals develop secondary-progressive MS; this is a form of the disease which progresses more steadily over time but involves fewer acute attacks and periods of remission. Nor is there a need to mention that there is yet another form of the disease called primary progressive MS which affects approximately one out of every ten patients diagnosed. This is a far more serious form of the disease with attacks that are rare and characterized by symptoms that gradually worsen over time. Forget about mentioning there is yet another form of the disease called progressive-relapsing MS where individuals develop worsening symptoms almost immediately upon being diagnosed and do not typically recover after each relapse.

All of this is way too complicated to even get into, so I choose to use the simple "frayed wire" analogy. I knew I should have applied to Harvard Medical School!

My only regret is that I did not get to tell my mom that I had MS before she passed away in 2009. I justify it by saying things like "There was no need to worry her," or "She wouldn't understand," or "I was fine." Truth is though that I should have told her. But I know today she is looking down and watching over me, spewing out constant reminders to "Take your medicine," and asking daily, "How are you feeling?" And of course, as a newspaper article junkie, she would have probably clipped and saved every article she came across that mentioned MS and given them to me whenever I'd see her. And, she probably would have played and won on a daily lottery number with the date of my diagnosis!

"Don't worry mom, I'll be fine!"

As I share my story with others, I tell people that "I am lucky" because people that have MS are impacted differently and have varying and more severe degrees of impairment. In some people, the wires that carry messages to different parts of the body are damaged, like the wires that go to the eyes, the lower and upper limbs, the portion of the brain dealing with memory or cognition, the bowel or bladder, etc. Some people with MS experience spasticity (which does affect me at times), have trouble seeing, have double vision, experience tingling sensations in their arms and legs, have great difficulty walking, have impaired speech or weakened memory, suffer with bowel or bladder urgency or incontinency issues, experience pain, etc. I'm fortunate at this point, as only my left leg is significantly impacted, my balance is at times off and bladder voiding/urgency peeks through the window (and my pants) on occasion. I guess the good guys got full after munching their way through my leg wires and decided it was time to take a break, have a cup of coffee and digest. I hope they go on a permanent diet never get hungry again!

I have gotten accustomed to withholding information from others about how I am feeling. I tend to not complain about my fatigue, my intolerance to heat, my bladder and balance issues, etc. I don't want to hear myself complain and burden others with my tales of woe, so I have stopped wearing long sleeved shirts a few years back. This helps me to not "wear my MS on my sleeve." But I do consider myself fortunate, as my eyes, mind, upper extremities, etc. are fine—at least for now. (But, my handwriting has gotten worse and does suck. But then again, it was never that great anyway)!

I thank the Lord that my cognitive abilities have not been impaired, as that's the one area which I rely on daily. Those who I tell about my affliction usually feel bad, saying things like "If you ever need anything, please let me know." I do not dwell on the fact that MS is a progressive disease and that it is likely to slowly worsen over time. But then again, it could stabilize and not get worse at all. As this is too much information to share and would likely lead to more inquiries and questions from others, I stop talking about it. I quickly change the subject so as not to elaborate any further, unless specifically asked. And besides, it is nobody's business. Only time will tell!

As time has gone on and I have opened up and told more people about my MS, disclosure has become easier. The tearing in my eyes and the crackling in my voice has all but disappeared. I have come to realize that things could be a lot worse and I have gone from asking "Why me?" to "Why *not* me?" (Yes, there are those days when I get so frustrated, feel so inadequate and get so pissed off that I let out a loud "This sucks—why has this happened to *me?*"). I would not be normal if I didn't. Of course, I'm careful that no one is within "ear shot" when I do rant and yell.

Don't get me wrong, to this day coping with my MS diagnosis and telling others still is not easy for me. I guess it never will be easy. I cannot wait for the day when I can tell people: "Yeah, I used to have this disease called Multiple Sclerosis that impacted my ability to walk and maintain my balance. But now, there is this medicine which I take every morning that helps restore and maintain my functionality, and there is another pill that I also take once a day in the afternoon that keeps my immune system in check and prevents the good cells from becoming 'hungry' and going on a ravenous attack. And today, I'm back to normal. Wanna race?"

Remaining optimistic for the future is what it is all about! There will come a day when functionality will be restored to all those suffering from MS. Having a positive attitude and an upbeat outlook is absolutely critical. It keeps me plowing ahead, and it gives me something to look forward to. Being optimistic and staying positive helps, *trust me*!

At present, nobody knows precisely what causes this disease of the central nervous system. It affects about 2.3 million people worldwide and approximately 450,000 people in the United States. Its severity ranges dramatically from person to person, from cases that are relatively benign to cases which are devastatingly disabling and bring either partial or complete paralysis to the body. These actual numbers may in fact be higher, as there likely are a good number of individuals who have the disease who have not yet been formally diagnosed due in large part to the invisible nature of the illness. MS can be as mysterious as it is complex and debilitating.

I decided to write this book and share my story in order to provide information and offer some inspiration to others by helping them to better cope with this horrible disease, and potentially inspire individuals to "get checked out" as soon as possible when they are just not feeling right. As my early symptoms were relatively minor and virtually non-existent, I shrugged-off my benign feelings/symptoms and attributed them to just getting older. Truthfully, I really *did* feel fine and it was only on rare occasions that I felt "off." But hindsight is 2020, so I strongly encourage everyone to listen to their bodies (and their spouse), and see a doctor ASAP when something just doesn't feel or seem right. Thank goodness my wife Luisa was persistent in her calls for me to see a physician and get checked-out. I guess she got tired of seeing me trip over my own two feet!

Perhaps if I had seen a doctor earlier, things may have turned out differently. There is a possibility that an earlier diagnosis may have resulted, and that I probably would have started treatments sooner. This may or may not have changed things; I guess I'll never know. But to all those reading this, I say: "Why wait and run the risk. Get checked out by a doctor!"

Just remember, whatever the situation, do not dwell in self-pity; I constantly remind myself of this. Get up, stand tall and dust yourself off (as difficult as this may be at times). Yes, "Why me?" is a common question to ask when confronted with a disturbing diagnosis like MS. But, just remember that God does not discriminate. You just need to make the best of your situation, channel your energies into a positive direction and remember: Things could be a lot worse! Consider yourself fortunate that something more dreadful has not appeared at your doorstep. And, should the MS doorbell ever ring for you (and I hope it never does), just pause for a moment to reflect before you answer. Sure, at first you'll be pissed off, be angry and upset and probably punch a wall or two. And of course, wonder and ask yourself, "Why is this happening to me?" These are normal initial reactions and emotions to have. But after a few days when you have had an opportunity to digest the information, take a deep breath, step back, reflect and calmly think to yourself, "Why _not_ me?"

My purpose for writing this book is simple: To share my story with others in the hopes of helping to increase awareness, put a common face behind this illness and give those diagnosed and living with MS some insights as to how I have been dealing with this awful disease. The unpredictable nature of the disease may have something do with the irregular and arbitrary manner in which I approach things. And at times, I feel saddened and become pensive. While I am sure that my actions have not always been perfect and worth emulating, they are genuine. If having MS has taught me anything, it has allowed me to shrug off 'the little things' in life that may have previously bothered me. When Lusia or anyone else gets upset about things others may say or do (like the driver who cuts you off on the road, or the motorist who does forty miles per hour in the left lane of the highway, or the person at the supermarket checkout line who nonchalantly removes items from their cart and presents them to the cashier in "slow motion," etc.), I often respond with something like "it's no big deal," or "don't worry about it" or "take it easy" or "yelling will not change anything." At times, I'm sure my carefree "what difference does it make" attitude gives Luisa and others the feeling that I do not care or have no sense of urgency about things; and I know it must frustrate them. In reality though, I have more or less adopted a "happy-go-lucky" outlook toward most things, realizing that it isn't until you are faced with a life-altering event like MS that you truly realize that it is not worth sweating the little things. Sure, those "little things" may have different meanings and greater levels of importance to different people. But, my having MS has helped me develop a higher level of tolerance in dealing with many daily events and issues. In a nutshell, everything is relevant and the "small stuff" is just not worth fretting about. "Life is too short." It is a shame that it takes a life altering event like an MS diagnosis to come to this realization!

So, I just keep *s'myelin* and move on!

Throughout this book, much of the dialogue has been reconstructed from memory, which means that in some cases quotes may or may not be word-for-word - so excuse some of the quotation marks. My intentions are not to misquote anyone; however, the essence of what I say is accurate. So for those people reading this who say, "I don't recall saying that," I will tell you that I have very distinct memories of these key interactions and have done my best to represent them to the best of my ability. I apologize for any perceived inexactitudes.

And now, here's my story...

Chapter 1

Vacationing in Italy

Vacation. Wow, I could not wait! After starting a new job at Credit Suisse in July 2003, I was ready for the calendar to turn to the second week of August in 2004 and gear myself up for the eight hour plane ride to Italy. Because of work commitments, I stayed behind in New York one additional week as my family traveled ahead. I remember leaving from John F. Kennedy (JFK) International Airport late on a Friday afternoon in early August; I was genuinely excited to be going on vacation. I kept myself occupied at the airport thinking about the oodles of study and reading materials I brought with me for the Series 7 Licensed Securities examination which I was scheduled to take at the end of the following month in September. Unfortunately, I was easily distracted and found ample excuses to not study like reading the newspaper, flipping through magazines that I had bought, purchasing M&Ms and candy bars to munch on, watching CNN on the overhead television screens in the JFK waiting area at the gate, people watching, etc. Anything but study! After all, I was starting a two week vacation and had plenty of time to study and review the materials on the airplane, at least that's what I kept telling

1

myself. Besides, I had never before flown Swiss Air, and that was something new that I was looking forward to.

On the long overnight airplane ride from New York to Italy, I admittedly did more sleeping than studying. But heck, I was starting vacation and was so anxious to arrive at my destination in Italy. Like I did in the airport before boarding the flight, I kept telling myself that I had plenty of time for studying. Flying Swiss Air was a slightly above average experience, and was really nothing special. Once on board the airplane, I sat in a window seat, ate typical airline food, read from my book, dozed-off at times or just relaxed. So much studying for the Series 7 exam (for now, anyway), and so much for the excitement and very high expectations I had for flying Swiss Air.

So after reading a bit from my book (*Leadership*, by Rudolph Giuliani) and sleeping for most of the flight over, I finally arrived early the next morning at Leonardo da Vinci airport in Rome. I de-boarded the plane, grabbed from the baggage claim area the two big pieces of luggage which I had checked, and navigated my way through the airport to find a train that would take me on the three hour ride to Abruzzi. Not speaking Italian made things more difficult for me, but I was able to manage and find my way to the right railway track. It took me a while though, but I got by. I should have plastered the phrase 'Mi Scusi, non parlo Italien molto biene" ("Excuse me, I do not speak Italian very well") on my forehead, as I said it so many times. All in all, I made it to my destination – not bad for a non-English speaking "Guido" from New York!

My destination was the Province of Chieti in Abruzzi, a small town in Italy about forty miles northwest of San Tomasso, the tiny mountain village where I'd be staying. San Tomasso was about three and one-half hours east of Rome and the town that my wife's parents came from. My wife (Luisa) and my daughters (Deanna and Lauren) had been there the entire week before, and they were looking forward to seeing me (I think).

After a two and one half hour plus train ride from Rome, I arrived at my final destination in Chieti. This is where Luisa, Deanna and Lauren came to pick me up with the car they had rented upon their arrival in Italy the week before. I remember the train pulling into the station around 3 P.M., fetching my two large suitcases and proceeding to disembark. I also remember the bags being heavy and clumsy and presenting me with a temporary challenge as I gathered and carried them off the train. In hindsight, I guess I struggled a bit; I paused for a brief moment to compose myself and then continued. Everything seemed just fine. Alas, there were three smiling faces waiting for me that were holding handmade "Welcome to Italy" signs, no less! I guess they were happy to see me after all.

After the long journey from New York, I was very tired and exhausted. This was despite the fact that I had slept during most of the flight over. I was looking forward to arriving in San Tomasso, unpacking, taking a hot shower and maybe grabbing a short nap. The final leg of my journey was about a fifty minute car ride from Chieti. I could not wait to arrive in San Tomasso; funny, because the "house" at which we would be staying was simple and tiny (a small four-room concrete structure, which was all of about 1,200 square feet in size and was the birthplace of my mother-in law). Don't get me wrong though. While small, it was very clean and uncluttered. It's just that when you mention to people that you're staying at a house in the mountains that your mother-in-law has in Italy, they automatically think of a villa in Tuscany. In contrast, our temporary residence in San Tomasso for the next six days consisted of a small kitchen with a tiny wash room and shower on the first floor, and two tiny bedrooms upstairs. Granted, this was not the Taj Mahal, but it was "home"—or would be *home* to me for the next week or so. It was, however, very nice, comfortable and welcoming, and would serve as my "Taj" throughout the stay. Long, hot showers were not the norm here (the small hot water tank supplied less than twenty minutes of "pleasure" for any given hour or so). Since I was always the last one to shower, I would take what I could get whenever I could. Finally though, I was "home" at last!

The next morning and for each of the next several days, Luisa and I would awaken promptly around 6:30 A.M. to the sounds of roosters crowing and the smell of pigs and other livestock that roamed the tiny streets and fields outside. We didn't need an alarm clock, and I don't even think we brought one with us anyway. Deanna and Lauren were oblivious to nature's "rise and shine" wake-up calls, and remained in deep slumbers until we shook and awakened them each morning around 9 A.M. After the girls were done "waking up" and washing, we all sat at the kitchen table downstairs and had breakfast. The cool, crisp fresh morning mountain air was extremely invigorating and the absence of a house telephone, cable TV and established cell phone signals was very refreshing (granted though, this took about a day or so to get used to). No emails, no ringing telephones, no text messages, no internet and no flipping through greater than one-hundred cable television channels (there were only four working channels on the small five inch black and white television set that sat on a corner cabinet across from the kitchen table at the Taj, with all the stations broadcast in Italian). The best thing was that there were no infomercials! There were no conference calls with work, no emails I had to wade through and no one calling from the office with work related questions. WOW! This was paradise! The absence of these things was replaced with the constant fight over bathroom usage, pleas that I made to the girls to not use *all* the hot water when showering, the smell of pigs and other livestock that permeated the air outside each morning, the herds of sheep being led by shepherds at sunset each evening and the hot August afternoons being in a house in Italy without air conditioning (outside, it would generally rise to nearly one-hundred degrees Fahrenheit by 3 P.M. each day). But, being up in the mountains in a small house encased in concrete made battling the hot August afternoons quite bearable. These were the big "challenges" we now faced. I couldn't remember having taken so many cold showers in my lifetime, and there were still nearly six days left to go! Always being the last one to shower, I got accustomed very quickly to the cold water, as the hot water tank was virtually fully depleted when it was my turn to clean up. But then again, beggars can't be choosy.

Each day the four of us would venture out to another small town. We were on the road and out and about by 10 A.M. and back to the Taj by 2 P.M. or so, just in time to join the locals who were taking their afternoon siestas. Sometimes we would take cover inside the "Taj" from the blistering sun and heat, or I would just relax on a hammock outside the house under a big shady tree. There were so many open air markets, shops and outdoor pizza and gelato stands that we saw and frequented. Upon our return to the house each day, there were some afternoons when we would also stop by and visit with many distant family members on my wife's side (cousins, I guess). These "cousins" were always begging us to stay for dinner, putting out wine and cheese, making espresso coffee and serving pizzelles, cookies and other homemade baked Italian delights, etc. Everyone's hospitality was pure. I quickly learned that everyone was a "cousin," even if they were not related. By the end of each visit, my face would hurt from smiling so much. My wife spoke Italian and would engage in conversations with them, as would Deanna and Lauren to a lesser degree; they would utilize the Italian language speaking skills they were learning in school. Me, on the other hand— _nothing._ Other than picking up a few random words here and there (and being fluent in some bad Italian curse words that were inappropriate to use), my Italian language skills were nonexistent, or "niente," as you might say. So, I'd sit, eat cheese, drink wine and smile a lot!

Each afternoon when we went back to "home base," I would join in with the traditional Italian custom of taking a siesta. Stretching out in a hammock or lounge chair under a big shade tree on the veranda out front to the side of the house, I would quickly doze off. I guess the homemade red wine everyone eagerly gave to me during our midday visits (or "rocket fuel" as I referred to it), did the trick. The cheese, Italian sausage, cookies and other homemade Italian pastries didn't hurt either. Boy, did I snooze. Now this was what vacation was all about; just relax and do nothing!

Around 7 P.M. each evening, Luisa, Deanna, Lauren and I would venture out to dinner after showering. We would generally hit a different eatery every night, and the food we found just got better and better with each new restaurant we visited. It seemed that all the restaurants referred to us by Luisa's distant relatives and family friends (the "cousins") were small out-of-the-way "mom-and-pop" establishments that many of which required you to walk through the kitchen upon entry in order to get to the main dining area. And after finishing each meal, the husband and wife owners of the restaurant would usually pull up chairs and sit at the table, engage in conversation with us (at least with Luisa, Deanna and Lauren who could understand and speak Italian), and offer us a whole series of desserts and after dinner cordials. Me? I would just grin, nod my head and smile. And oh yeah, I'd never pass-up eating those tasty desserts! There was one restaurant close by to San Tomasso called La Tana Del Lupo that offered outdoor seating that we enjoyed and went to a few times. Almost always, the owners of the "small-town" restaurants would talk about brothers of aunts or uncles who had third cousins with siblings once removed, whose parents had married children with one spouse that was a distant relative of Luisa's family, etc. Whew! The nice thing about this small Italian town was that everybody seemed to know everybody, and had some sort of lineage with Luisa's mom or dad. Deanna and Lauren loved the attention and couldn't wait for the tartuffe, homemade ice cream and gelato to be brought out for dessert. And neither could I! Now this was awesome!

Each evening after dinner, we would arrive home at the Taj around 10 P.M. and would congregate in the small kitchen with neighbors, and of course with the many "cousins." Out would come the homemade red wine, cheese, Italian sausage, cookies, etc. Deanna and Lauren would venture upstairs to bed shortly afterwards by this point in the evening. Each night was capped off with what seemed like endless cups of black espresso coffee. And of course, there was the homemade limoncello! After everyone left, usually by midnight, Luisa would turn in and I would stay downstairs in the kitchen, break out the books, my laptop computer and study materials I had brought across the ocean with me to study for the upcoming Series 7 exam. Most nights, I put in about three or four hours, generally retiring around 3:00 A.M.-ish. I guess I was feeling guilty about slouching, sleeping and not studying on the airplane ride over, so I "burned the midnight oil." Reading about municipal bonds, warrants, option straddles, etc. at the kitchen table in Italy was _not_ a lot of fun, but it was something I had to do. Thank goodness for the red wine and limoncello that initially mellowed me out, followed by the countless cups of espresso that kept me wired, fully awake and allowed me to study until about 3 A.M. each night. I was so wide awake that I couldn't even go to sleep if I wanted to.

After spending six days in San Tomasso, it was time to leave and depart for Rome in order to shop and sightsee. We said our arrivedercis to the people in the town the night before, as we made our rounds to about eight or ten homes and said goodbye to about thirty or forty "cousins." I could swear we said goodbye to the entire population of San Tomasso (which we probably did). My cheeks and my torso were sore from all the kissing and hugging. Throughout our visit, everyone was so nice and kind. But now, it was time to leave this carefree and stress-free existence. I often wonder if the people who live in Italy have it right and us here in America have the wrong priorities. Whatever, it was now time to move on.

The next morning, we awoke at 4 A.M. to get an early start on our three-plus hour car ride to Rome. By the time we got to the autostrada, Deanna and Lauren were fast asleep. Hard to believe that we were traveling nearly ninety miles per hour and that most cars were still passing us! We made one or two stops along the way on the autostrada at the auto-grille for coffee and bathroom breaks.

Rome. What a great city. I remember driving up to a small, quaint little hotel Luisa and I found online when planning the trip that was just right across from the Spanish Steps. I was glad to have the hotel attendants take the car and park it, since driving in the city of Rome was challenging, to say the least. We arrived around noon the first day, and after unpacking and getting a quick bite to eat, we casually made our way outside the hotel to explore our new surroundings. After having dinner and retiring early the first day, we would regularly awaken early each of the following mornings, typically around 8 A.M., grab breakfast at the hotel (usually croissants, pastries and coffee) and head out. Most days were spent strolling down the many streets and stopping in the countless stores. The kids loved walking along the Via Veneto (Rome's version of New York City's 5th Avenue), and stopping in the many stores. Most were designer shops like Fendi, Gucci, Ferragamo, Bruno Magli, etc. I'm not a big shopper, but I tagged along and was a good citizen. And besides, I had something they needed; the credit card!

Wow, was it hot in Rome! It was at least ninety degrees Fahrenheit each day throughout our five day stay! And of course, it felt so much hotter as we walked around the large, crowded city in the middle of August. Thank goodness for bottles of cold 'aqua fesca' (water) and gelato! I'm glad I experienced Rome when I did, as today I would not have been able to do the walking and tolerate the oppressive heat and humidity.

Each day seemed to be more hot and humid than the day before, so I welcomed the many times when we would stop inside a cold, air conditioned store. Our excursions past countless shops resulted in more window shopping than buying, but it was fun nonetheless. Of course, we would stop repeatedly at the many outdoor cafes for some cold water, pizza and gelato. After returning to our hotel in the late afternoons for much needed showers (at least this time, I didn't have to worry about the absence of hot water and the need to take a cold shower) and occasionally take a short nap, we would venture out again early each evening to a nice restaurant (usually one that was recommended by someone at the hotel's front desk). And at night, at least it was cooler outside than it was during the daytime. Still though, we needed air conditioning when we retired back to our hotel room each evening.

One night we dined with Patrick Coon and his wife Alison. Patrick was a senior executive on assignment in Utah at one of the vendors I interfaced with when I worked for Credit Suisse back in the states. Patrick and Alison, who lived back in the state of Texas, were celebrating their twenty-fifth wedding anniversary with a vacation to Rome. I remember chatting with Patrick in his office in Salt Lake City earlier in the year, and we mused about how we would be vacationing in Italy during the month of August and that we would be in Rome on the exact same days. We promised we would contact one another while in Rome and plan to get together for dinner one evening. So, true to our word, we hooked up and made plans to meet.

While in Rome and seeing Patrick and Alison one night, we were waiting to be seated at a restaurant for dinner. I recall perching myself up against a small ledge to rest as we chatted with the Coons and waited for a table. I was sure all the walking we did earlier that day, combined with the extreme heat and humidity, was seeking revenge on me. It was the first time I had interfaced socially with Patrick, and the first time we had met one another's respective spouses. Shortly after arriving at the restaurant and waiting for a table, we were seated and enjoyed a fabulous dinner. I remember Patrick and I commenting when the check arrived about how inexpensive the dinner was (at least compared to U.S. prices) considering the plentiful portions of food we had, its high quality and the two bottles of red wine that we enjoyed. After dinner, we all took a stroll around the city. After stopping for gelato, we arrived at the Spanish Steps and walked to the top. True to form, mid-way up the steps clumsy me tripped and spilled my cup of gelato all over me. I was wearing a brand-new polo shirt too—what a mess! We all laughed, and of course Luisa called me an awkward and clumsy "xxx" [*clod*]. We then continued strolling the streets of Rome as if nothing happened. I'm sure if I were to trip climbing stairs and spill something today, no one would laugh or say anything aside from expressing concern about my wellbeing. Oh well.

The Coons—what a wonderful couple! We all hit it off really well, and enjoyed a fabulous dinner (and for a while, some gelato too)! To this day, we remain good friends with Patrick and Alison, having traveled once to their home in Dallas and having once hosted them at our summer home in East Hampton. We also interact with them frequently via e-mail and on Facebook, and remain abreast of what is happening with one another's families.

Then it was back to the hotel. Everyone was dead tired from all the walking we did and the day's extreme heat, and quite full from stuffing ourselves from dinner and dessert. Except for me, everybody went right to sleep. Me, on the other hand, I grabbed my books and my laptop, sat out on the lit hotel patio outside our room and studied/did practice exams preparing for the following month's Series 7 examination. I studied until around 4 A.M. that night, something I did for each of the remaining nights while on vacation in Rome. Yes, I was *very* tired, but I was *very* determined to pass that exam! (Oh, and by the way, I did pass the exam, scoring an 84)!

Our last three days in Rome were spent mostly sightseeing (the Coliseum, Saint Peter's Basilica, Vatican City, the Trevi Fountain, etc.).

We also sprinkled-in some window shopping. The Coliseum was magnificent and the Trevi Fountain was cool (literally), but nothing topped Vatican City. It amazes me how one man (Michelangelo) could lay on his back and intricately craft such a fine work of art on that ceiling, the Sistine Chapel. I have difficulty painting a ceiling with a roller, and get dizzy just thinking about it. Incredible!

While at Vatican City, I distinctly remember walking with Lusia, Deanna and Lauren down a long set of wide and curvy marble stairs. There was a picture posted along the stairway route (similar those blue handicap signs you see in the United States that are posted in malls and public places), of a harried stick figure person. A big circle and a slash went across the placard signifying "No Running," or "non in esecuzione." We all stopped and laughed, with Luisa and the girls saying that the uncoordinated and stumbling stick figure on the sign reminded them of me. In fact, I remember Luisa, Deanna and Lauren each insisting that I pose in front of the sign to have my picture taken. Wow, how ironic. Who knew?

After having spent a splendid two weeks in Italy, it was time to come home and venture back to reality in the USA. Off we flew from Leonardo da Vinci airport in Rome leaving a wonderful set of memories behind. In some respects, we were all very anxious to return home. In other respects, I continued to wonder if the stress free, relaxed manner in which the locals of Italy lived wasn't a healthier and more enhanced lifestyle compared to what we have in the states. Once on the airplane, each of us "collapsed" and nodded off from what was a very active and fun-filled vacation.

And so, eight hours later we landed and arrived in New York City at JFK. The crowds, the hustle, the bustle, the multitude of languages that were spoken, the general lack of courtesy most of the people had, etc. was surely a stark reminder that we were "home." Thoughts about the calm, laid-back culture in Italy would often resonate in my mind

11

after returning to work the following Monday. But, after a few short days, my vacation to Italy was just a distant memory. Impromptu conference calls, the hectic and stressful existence of a Wall Street trading floor and working late nights once again became the normal routine. I really do miss those afternoon Italian siestas!

In hindsight, I am so happy I made this trip to Italy in 2004. All the walking, the extreme heat and the constant running-around would certainly make a similar trip less likely for me today.

The next year or so was relatively routine for me. I traveled for business a fair amount of the time (mainly to California, Salt Lake City Utah, Dallas Texas, Fort Mill North Carolina and Jacksonville Florida), and put in my share of late nights. The job I had started at Credit Suisse in July 2003 was going well and gave me the opportunity to deal with a number of challenging situations. Other than maybe one or two very isolated stumbles, I was fine. Then, in November 2005 some strange things started to happen.

Chapter 2

Vacuuming the Lawn

It was the middle of November 2005 and Luisa and I had just purchased from Sears a heavy duty lawn vacuum to help with picking up the leaves that had fallen across the property at our vacation home in East Hampton. Having built the house in the year 2000, we still remained somewhat fanatical five years later about doing everything we could to keep our home looking as pristine as possible, and manicuring the lawn was no exception. We were proud of the fact that we were able to purchase the floor model of the lawn vacuum that was on display at the Hicksville store, as Sears was out of stock and indicated there was a two-week lead time before the item would again be available and delivered to the store. The salesperson at Sears swore by the machine and said that it not only did a great job picking up the leaves and twigs, but that it left the lawn looking very neat and freshly manicured. (We later learned that he was absolutely right)! He said that since this was the only such machine that remained in the store, we had a choice of either taking the floor model, seeing if one was available for pick-up at another Sears store or waiting two weeks for delivery to the Hicksville store when the new stock arrived. He went on to tell us that he could probably get us a good deal if we took the floor model. He excused himself and walked away to check (I assume with a store manager or a supervisor). After about five minutes, he returned to the area we were standing at and told us that he could sell us the floor model for four hundred-fifty dollars plus tax. Fantastic! That would allow us to save an additional eighty-nine dollars off the regular sales price of five hundred thirty-nine dollars, and we would *not* have to wait. We jumped at the offer and decided to take the floor model for four hundred-fifty dollars, plus tax "As Is." We did clarify with the sales-person however, that should we find anything wrong with the machine or decided we no longer wanted it, we could return it for a full refund. Since it was a floor model, we wanted to be absolutely sure before pur-chasing it. Besides, saving a fair amount of money and having it avail-able for immediate use was a *huge* benefit associated with purchasing the floor model. Plus, we would *not* need to spend time assembling it! The only problem we thought we'd have would be getting the large, bulky machine into the car. Thank goodness we had a big Toyota Se-quoia Sport Utility Vehicle (SUV). After paying, a store clerk rolled the machine to the rear of the store where we had moved the car. After a few twists and turns and removing the two screws that held the push bar on top of the unit, we loaded the machine into the Sequoia for transport and were on our way.

We were very excited to get the machine as quickly as possible and begin "vacuuming." Ecstatic to have saved nearly one-hundred dollars by purchasing the assembled floor model, we were quite relieved that we did not need to fork over five-hundred dollars to a gardener for a fall leaf and twig clean-up. Besides, we knew a gardener would not have done the same quality job that we would do. In one season, this machine will have paid for itself, and no assembly was required! Can't beat that! In the next three or four years that followed, the machine would get a full workout each fall, as we did the clean-up ourselves. (By 2010 though, pushing the vacuum and emptying the bag had become too much for me to handle, and was also too much for Luisa to deal with as well). So the following year, it would be back to forking over dough to a gardener to perform the fall clean-up. For several years that followed, the vacuum sat idle in the corner of my garage in East Hampton. In 2014, I wound up giving the machine to my brother-in-law Tony so at least he could use it at his home in Howard Beach, Queens. Amazingly, after several years of not using it and having it sit idle and filled with gasoline, Tony was able to start the machine right up on the first try. It worked beautifully! Afterwards, he did however, change the oil and replace the carburetor as a precaution. Remarkably, the vacuum looked brand new.

It was a cold crisp Friday morning in the middle of November, 2005. After loading the machine we had purchased from Sears into our SUV, we drove from our primary residence in Jericho out to our secondary home in Suffolk County, East Hampton. We stopped along the way for some pizza and a quick rest room break for the girls, and then quickly got back on the road and resumed driving. We could not wait to get to the house, fill the machine with gasoline and begin our landscaping work. It was nice to be so young and so eager. Can you imagine, looking forward to doing yardwork? After driving nearly ninety miles, we approached a gas station in the Hamptons and filled a five gallon plastic container that we purchased from Sears with gas; $2.29 per gallon! (Had I thought about it before, I would have stopped for gas near our home in Nassau County and paid the _bargain_ price of $1.99 per gallon). After filling the container with gas in the Hamptons, we then drove the short distance to our house.

We arrived at our home in East Hampton early that Friday afternoon and quickly unloaded the vacuum from the Sequoia, re-attached the push bar, filled it with the gasoline we had purchased that was in the container, mixed it with the oil that came with our purchase, pulled the starter cord (a few times) and—VOILA! We were vacuuming! We were so excited that we didn't even go inside upon our arrival at the house (although Deanna and Lauren did). If I'm not mistaken, we probably didn't even bother to close the lift gate on the Sequoia until well later in the afternoon. As soon as we arrived at the house, Luisa and I went right to work. The machine gobbled up and mulched the leaves, small twigs and dead grass, and within twenty minutes the attached burlap bag was filled with nearly twenty pounds of debris! Wow, this was great. The salesperson at Sears was spot on when he said that the machine would leave the lawn looking very neat and manicured. This was evidenced by the tiny piece of lawn that we had cleaned so far. Only .99 acres to go!

What we had done thus far looked great, and it felt wonderful to be out in the crisp forty-five degree air and see such progress. It was a bright, sunny day, with no wind; perfect weather to be outdoors working. It was a beautiful fall day indeed. After a number of passes over the front lawn were complete and the vacuum bag became filled, the big burlap "catcher" bag needed to be unhooked from the machine, carried to the back of the house and emptied. That was my job, to unfasten the bag, carry/drag it across to the rear of the property and empty its contents into the wooded reserve area bordering the house. Then, it was back to the front of the house where it was time to reattach the bag and begin the vacuuming process all over again. At first, this process did not seem like work at all. It was actually a lot of fun. We could not believe how perfectly manicured the lawn looked for the sections we had completed. After about forty minutes or so and a few passes made by Luisa across the lawn with the machine, I convinced Luisa to let me try and vacuum for a while. She agreed (reluctantly, as she was having too much fun), and handed me the reins, but only for a few minutes. For this go-'round, once the bag was filled (which by the way I was still tasked with unhooking, carrying and emptying it into the woods), my turn vacuuming was over. Then it was back to our primary roles: Luisa as "Vacuumer-In-Chief" and me as "Captain of Waste Disposal."

Seeing the cleared and manicured lawn paths across our front yard was quite gratifying, and the lawn truly looked great! But, after making about ten trips or so, we both realized this was not that easy, and that it was actually hard "work." Plus, on or about the tenth trip I made to carry/drag the bag across the lawn and dump the contents in the reserve area in the rear of the property, I had to lean against a tree for a brief moment before walking back to the front of the house. I found this necessary in order to catch my breath and "recharge my batteries." I became fatigued and my legs felt heavy and weak, at least temporarily. Then, it was back to the front lawn to begin the routine all over again. After a short rest between detaching, emptying and re-attaching the bag, I was good to go for another ten or so rounds. I followed this routine on a consistent basis, and I'd take a short "rest" on about every tenth or twelfth trip. At one point, Luisa saw me resting and yelled out, saying amusingly: "Hey, no sitting down on the job. There's plenty of work to do!" We both laughed and just kept working. Toward the end of the day, I was taking a break to "recharge my batteries" on about every sixth or seventh trip, and no longer carried the bag to the rear of the house. Instead, I began dragging it. I thought nothing of my tiredness, the heavy feeling in my legs and the need to rest momentarily after emptying the bag and dumping the leaves. "Hey, I must be getting old," I thought to myself. Throughout the day, it was common to see deer running across the property, particularly when the machine was shut down and turned off between bag disposals. But once we started up the machine again and resumed working, the sound of the motor must have scared the deer away and they were nowhere to be found. I'm sure that they were watching us from afar, antlers raised and smiling!

Lusia and I worked until dusk that Friday, realizing that tomorrow was another day and more "clean-up" of the leaf covered lawn awaited us. Now almost night time, we decided to quit and call it a day. What we had done thus far looked great, and although we were tired, we looked forward to getting back to work very early the next day. The lawn area in front and on the sides of the entire house was done, and it looked phenomenal! After closing the lift gate on the Sequoia and heading inside the house to wash-up, we enjoyed a nice dinner with Deanna and Lauren that Luisa pulled together. To say Luisa and I had hearty appetites was an under-statement. I guess working outdoors on a crisp fall day made us very hungry! After dinner, we both turned-in. Boy, did we sleep well that night!

The next morning was Saturday, and boy did it seem to come early. After we had breakfast, we immediately resumed work at around 7 A.M. vacuuming the lawn, this time in the rear of the house. Before we started to work, I went to the filling station to fill our red plastic gas can with more fuel. We were ready to go and resume work. On this day, I recall resting on average after every fifth or sixth trip I made to detach and empty the burlap bag. On maybe a dozen or so occasions, Luisa let me "hold the reins" and work the machine. I'm sure this occurred mostly whenever Luisa needed a break. Even on those occasions when I commanded the machine, I was still responsible for detaching and emptying the bag's contents into the reserve. For the most part though, Luisa vacuumed while I used a rake to clean the leaves out of the bushes and those areas around the house where the machine could get to. After about ten hours (with only a short break for lunch and one or two bathroom breaks), our task was complete and the property looked great! The front lawn, side lawns and rear lawn were all done! Plus, we saved money and didn't need to fork anything over to a gardener, who by the way wouldn't have done nearly as good a job as we did! The machine we had just purchased two days earlier clearly paid for itself with one fall clean-up. It was around 5:00 P.M. and almost dark. We then cleaned-up and stored the vacuum and yard rakes in the garage, went inside the house, washed-up, ordered a pizza (which I drove into town to pick up) and sat down to eat. Both Luisa and I were tired and looked forward to just relaxing that evening and sleeping a little later the next morning before packing up and making the ninety-mile drive home. After our pizza dinner, Luisa and I both crashed on the couch in the living room. We watched television for a short while, and then retired to bed. Deanna and Lauren entertained themselves after dinner playing video games on the computer in the upstairs loft. Again, we slept like logs!

After we woke up around 10 A.M. the next morning, we grabbed some breakfast and gazed out at the lawn from the rear kitchen windows. We were so proud of the job we had done and were not shy about "patting ourselves on the back" and taking a bow. As we slowly walked the property, were overcome with joy and felt a huge sense of accomplishment! Even the deer, who welcomed the quietness since there was no longer a vacuum running, grazed across the picturesque landscape seeming to approve. Our neighbor Sal, walking his dog along the street in the front of our house, stopped and commented about how nice the property looked. Clearly, that was a welcome remark that just validated what we were thinking, that "we dun good!" Luisa and I were both very tired, but all the hard work paid-off and was well worth the effort. We joked about whether or not we should contact _Home & Garden Magazine_ to have them take pictures of the property and do a feature story about our home in an upcoming edition. The premises around the house really looked fantastic!

Later that Sunday in the early afternoon, we drove home. Again, I attributed my "tiredness" to my age and to being out of shape (wow, I turned all of forty-five earlier in March of that year). Having worked behind a desk at Citibank for the prior fifteen plus years was not exactly the type of conditioning needed for such a task. Plus, as the years passed by, Luisa and I were becoming more comfortable calling in vendors to handle small jobs (like interior painting, staining the deck, etc.). And my new role on the trading floor at Credit Suisse did not offer any further type of physical conditioning. Boy though, was I happy to hold a white color job. I could not fathom the thought of being employed in a vocation that required manual labor!

On the drive home, there were countless cries from Deanna and Lauren of "What took you so long?" and "Where were you all day yesterday?" and "Can we stop along the way home for ice cream?" These were typical chants and questions from eight and eleven-year-olds. In the back of my mind, I realized why gardeners charged so much for the fall clean-up task, and was convinced more than ever that the five-hundred-dollar investment we made in purchasing the machine was certainly a bargain! I'm sure Luisa was thinking the same thing. Heading back to work on Monday would seem like a welcome rest. I could not wait! Thanksgiving was approaching in a few days and it was only going to be a three-day work-week anyway. I was looking forward to resting and enjoying the upcoming Thanksgiving holiday and spending a nice four-day weekend with the family. No yardwork—just eating turkey, watching football, visiting with relatives and relaxing. And of course, watching reruns of the Twilight Zone and the Honeymooners! With Thanksgiving approaching I know my mom, dad and Luisa's mom would be happy to see us, especially seeing the kids.

As I think back, one thing seems strange now. I had done physical labor around the house and yard many times before in the past (i.e. leaf raking, fall and spring clean-ups, tree trimming, lawn mowing, planting shrubs, snow shoveling, power washing, painting, etc.). But after the weekend with the lawn vacuum, I remember being totally wiped out when the task was completed, and I slept "like a log" that first night home. The good news was that by the next morning, the alarm went off at 5:30 A.M. and I felt totally fine. As I showered, I thought to myself how glad I was that the next fall clean-up was another twelve months away! The money we had spent on the lawn vacuum was well worth it, as we had already recouped our investment.

For Thanksgiving, we ate by my mother-in-law's house in Howard Beach, Queens, but stopped first to visit my parents. We spent about an hour or so at their house in Richmond Hill, Queens, and my mom immediately asked, "Why are you limping?" She did kiss me first and wished me a Happy Thanksgiving. After ignoring and not answering the question, my mom asked again. Finally, I replied that I was not limping and she snapped back saying, "Don't tell me. I know you are limping!" I shrugged it off (largely because I felt I really was walking normally and was not limping at all). My mother was keenly astute! I enjoyed the remainder of my visit with my parents and after an hour or so, departed with Luisa, Deanna and Lauren to my mother-in-law's house in nearby Howard Beach to enjoy Thanksgiving dinner. My brother-in-law Tony joined us for dinner, and we had a splendid Thanksgiving feast. Afterwards, he and I relaxed on the couch and watched football (flipping channels during commercial breaks to view portions of _Twilight Zone_ episodes).

Chapter 3

You Don't Have Lyme Disease!

After putting it off and repeatedly telling myself there was nothing wrong with me, Luisa remained adamant that I see our doctor and get checked out. "You trip and stumble too often," she'd say, "and that heaviness in your legs is not normal. Even the kids have noticed that you stumble on occasion. You need to make an appointment to see the doctor." I listened, smiled and then joked. "So I'm clumsy, big deal. I was never that coordinated growing up anyway." Luisa, who was not laughing, reminded me: "True, you have been clumsy ever since I met you. But lately, you have been *very* clumsy, tripping over your own two feet and being all thumbs. Plus, you always complain that you're tired every night when you come home from work. You need to get checked out." I tried making light of her comments, but Luisa was not backing down. She reminded me again about the heaviness I felt in my legs when I was working in the yard and how I had to rest frequently to regain my strength. She also reminded me of the occasional trips and stumbles I had over the past six months or so when I was either walking in the mall or puttering around the house, and again mentioned to me how I was always complaining about feeling tired when I came home from work. I remember her getting annoyed at me for taking things so lightly and being so strong-headed about everything being fine and that there was no need to see the doctor. She said abruptly, "…Should I continue?" At this point, I knew she wasn't kidding around, so I thought it best to heed her advice and schedule an appointment to see our family doctor. I told her I needed to schedule an appointment anyway for my annual physical, and that I would be sure to mention everything to the doctor. After that, the discussion ended.

It was the first week of December 2005, and I was already two months overdue anyway to see my primary care physician Dr. Dilorenzo for my annual physical. So, just as I did each year prior (albeit two months late this time), I visited my primary care doctor and underwent a variety of routine tests; blood pressure, electro-cardiogram, urine analysis, bloodwork, prostate check (uugghh, how I hated the sound of that rubber glove snapping)!… all the routine things. I fasted from 11 P.M. the night before in anticipation of having bloodwork done. The next day, I arrived at the doctor's office at 10 A.M. and to put it mildly, was quite famished. The examination started with Dr. Dilorenzo's nurse drawing two vials of blood from me, checking my weight, height, blood pressure and giving me an electro cardiogram. I figured the electro cardiogram would take longer than it did but within a matter of less than five minutes, the test was complete. I recall having a cardiogram done many years ago and it then lasting what seemed like an eternity. I even joked to the nurse about how quick the test was, and she acknowledged that the procedure had been significantly streamlined over the years. Shortly after she was done and left the room, Dr. Dilorenzo came into the office to examine me.

I had been a patient of Dr. Dilorenzo for about ten years, and I swear he looked exactly the same as he did the first time I met him. Slim and fit with dark hair and always sporting an even tan, Dr. Dilorenzo was a middle aged man who, any time I would see him, sported a long white medical jacket. He had a friendly personality, was very easy-going and never rushed you out of his office. He was very easy to talk with. Generally speaking, he was a really "nice guy," whom I felt very comfortable with discussing any topic. Throughout the exam, I asked the usual questions of him—i.e. "Is my blood pressure normal?" "How's my heart?" "Electro Cardiogram okay?" "Does my urine look good?" "Prostate seem okay?" "Glands feel normal?" He took the time to answer all of my questions and assured me when he was done examining me that I should relax and that "everything looks just fine."

My visit with Dr. Dilorenzo took about thirty minutes. Toward the end of my appointment as he was about to leave the room and as I was putting my shirt back on, Dr. Dilorenzo asked if I had any other questions. I paused and almost said no, nothing else. _But I didn't._ In my mind, I knew that when I arrived home, the first thing Lusia would ask me was what the doctor said when you mentioned to him about your occasional stumbles, feeling tired most of the time and the heaviness you felt in your legs when you were cleaning up the leaves in the yard last month. I did not want to tell Luisa that I never raised it, so I figured I'd bring up the subject with Dr. Dilorenzo. And I did. As he was just about to exit the room, I called to stop him.

"Yeah, Doctor, there is one other thing I want to mention to you. Actually, there is something that my wife wants me to mention to you." With Dr. Dilorenzo's hand on the door knob and with him about to exit the room, I told him what Luisa had said: "My wife says that I'm clumsy and occasionally trip over my own two feet and that I should get checked out." Dr. Dilorenzo and I both chuckled and had a good laugh. He told me that wives typically say that their husbands are clumsy, and that it must be a "wife thing." Then, I mentioned to Dr. Dilorenzo the temporary heaviness I had felt in my legs as I was cleaning up the leaves in the yard, my need to rest between yardwork tasks, and the tired feeling that overcame me as that day progressed. I also told him that there were days after coming home from work that I would feel very tired. He stood at the doorway looking at me and listening. He then closed the door behind him, walked back into the room and pulled up a stool to sit on. He asked that I tell him more about the heaviness I had felt in my legs. I told him that I was doing a fall clean-up of the leaves at my house on the east end of Long Island in the Hamptons, and that I needed to rest every so often before continuing so that I could regain my strength. I also told him that I felt fatigued, that my legs felt tired and heavy most of the time after doing a stretch of yardwork, and remember thinking that I could not wait for it to get dark so that I could stop working, go inside the house and sit down on the couch to watch television and relax. I let him know that each time I felt like this, I would take a brief rest between rounds of performing yardwork for about two minutes or so to "recharge my batteries." After that, I remember telling him that I would feel fine again and was ready for "round two."

Dr. Dilorenzo listened to my story, and then immediately asked if I remembered recently getting any bug bites. I looked at him rather quizzically, as his question seemed somewhat odd to me. I thought for a moment and told him that nothing like that, other than a mosquito bite or two, came to mind. "Why?" I asked. He briefly paused, did not say anything or immediately respond to my question, and then looked down at my medical chart. Next, he did a quick scan of my arms (for bug bites, I guess), and talked about prescribing bloodwork for me in order to specifically check for Lyme disease. As he was examining my body, I remember him explaining that since the Hamptons had a considerable tick population due to the many deer that roamed about, he just wanted to be sure that I did not have any tick bites. He then further explained to me that Lyme disease was generally brought on by a tick bite. He reiterated to me that the Hamptons are loaded with deer, and that the woods are filled with ticks. He told me that several of his patients had contracted Lyme disease over the years after being out in the Hamptons, and because of that he did not want to take any chances.

"Lyme disease?" I asked." I've heard of it but am not exactly sure what it is." "Yes, Lyme disease," he said, "it's probably nothing, and I do not see any bug bites or scars on your arms. I just want to be sure, because if it is Lyme disease and it goes untreated, it can cause a variety of problems, including stumbling, chronic tiredness, joint aches and pains, heaviness in the legs, etc. These are some of the more common early symptoms. Since you have been experiencing some of these symptoms, it may be a good idea to run some bloodwork and check for Lyme disease. Longer term, untreated Lyme disease can cause neurological damage." I remember thinking that all the symptoms he described about Lyme disease were "spot on" to what I was experiencing, so therefore that must be what I had. As I thought some more, I said to myself, "Wow, neurological problems. That does not sound good!" To be absolutely certain, Dr. Dilorenzo wanted to take another look at my entire body, so I removed my shirt that I had put back on earlier at the end of my initial examination, and lowered my trousers as well. He did another more complete and thorough scan of my entire body, this time a bit slower. Dr. Dilorenzo's scan did not reveal any noticeable bug bites, let alone any bites that I may have gotten from a tick. He did, however, order the blood test for Lyme disease. I remember him saying that while he did not see anything, he was giving me a script nonetheless for bloodwork, "just to be sure." The doctor shook my hand, handed me a prescription ordering the bloodwork and asked if there was anything else. I said that at this time there was nothing else. He laughed, and we then said goodbye. I guess he was off to see the next patient. After he left the room and I was just about finished getting dressed, I thought I heard the sound of a rubber glove snap coming from the adjacent examination room. He must have been doing another prostate exam! When I finished getting dressed, I left the examination room and made my way out to the receptionist area. I then proceeded to give the office assistant/receptionist my co-payment, telling her that I would see her next year and went on my way. Driving home, I was starving because I had not eaten anything all morning, so I remember stopping to eat two slices of pizza for lunch.

When I came home from the doctor, Luisa immediately asked: "So, what did Dilorenzo say?" Good thing I had mentioned to him about my stumbling, tiredness and leg heaviness. "Nothing much," I said. "He says I look fine and that all my vitals seem good but that he wants to check for Lyme disease caused by a potential tick bite, so he ordered a special blood test." I again told her that he said that everything else looked good, and that he was ordering the blood test for Lyme disease just to be sure. I then told Luisa that the doctor seemed to get a bit more interested and focused when I mentioned to him that my fatigue and leg heaviness came about when I was doing yardwork out in the Hamptons. I told Luisa that Dr. Dilorenzo's interest had peaked because of all the deer that run around the Hamptons and the fact that they are known for carrying ticks. I also told Luisa what Dr. Dilorenzo had said, that several of his patients over the years had contracted Lyme disease that were caused from tick bites that they likely received from time they spent in the Hamptons. I then told her what the doctor had indicated; that some of the early symptoms of having Lyme disease included stumbling, tiredness, joint aches and pains, and heaviness in the legs. Luisa nodded her head and said, "It's good you're getting that bloodwork done then. See, I told you it might be something." She was glad to hear that I was getting checked out, and she reiterated what I had just said about all the deer running around the yard out east. "Relax," I said, "so I'll get the blood test. It's probably nothing." I nodded and smiled. The discussion was about to end, but not before Luisa mentioned one last thing: "Didn't your friend Jerry have Lyme disease at one point a few years ago?" she asked. "Yeah, I think so," I responded. Jerry has a summer house in

Hampton Bays, and did in fact get a tick bite that caused him to contract Lyme disease. I remember him complaining of joint aches and pains and feeling tired for several months, prompting him to eventually see a doctor. As I recall, he waited a few months before seeing a doctor and went undiagnosed for a short period. Prior to that time, he seemed to be chronically tired, lethargic and was experiencing joint pains for several months. Once it was confirmed that he had Lyme disease and he began taking antibiotics, it took Jerry several months thereafter for him to begin feeling better. Luisa and I spoke about this, and I remember saying to her, "So I guess what Dr. Dilorenzo says makes sense. I'll get my blood checked, just to be sure." From that point forward, there was no further discussion on the subject.

The next day was Saturday, and I drove to Quest Laboratories early that morning for the blood test. I think it took me more time to drive the couple of miles from my home to the lab than it actually took for me to take the blood test. I no sooner went into the lab and rolled-up my sleeve when the technician said he was all done after inserting the needle into my arm to draw blood. But my trip to the lab wasn't a total waste of time. On the way home, I stopped for gasoline, and then for bagels so that everyone could enjoy them for breakfast. Again, I was careful not to eat or drink anything prior to going for the bloodwork, so by the time I arrived home with the bagels I was starving.

The following Monday around mid-day, I called Dr. Dilorenzo's office for the results of the routine bloodwork performed during my annual physical. I figured that the results from the Lyme disease blood test I took on Saturday had not come back yet, but figured I'd ask anyway, just in case they did. After a brief hold, Dr. Dilorenzo came to the telephone and rattled off the following: "Urine, normal. Triglycerides, fine at 105. Vitamin D level, normal. PSA, great at .6. HDL (Good Cholesterol), excellent at 121. LDL (Bad Cholesterol), very good at 44. Everything looks perfect!" I also asked if he had gotten the results from the Lyme disease bloodwork (which I assumed he did not, but I asked nonetheless). Confirming what I thought, Dr. Dilorenzo said that the results for the Lyme disease bloodwork had *not* come back yet, and that I should call back his office for those results in another day. That Wednesday afternoon while at work, I called Dr. Dilorenzo's office late in the day. After being kept on hold for nearly five minutes, he came to the phone and said: "The blood test has come back negative," meaning that I *did not* have Lyme disease. I was somewhat relieved, but that relief quickly disappeared though when he next said, "....While you *don't* have Lyme disease, I'd like to refer you to the general neurologist I usually recommend patients see to be sure there isn't anything more serious going on." I gulped. Dr. Dilorenzo likely sensed the concern in my voice when I said, "Something more serious?" Realizing I was concerned, he told me, "It's probably nothing," but he then quickly said that he'd prefer if I saw his neurologist and got checked out anyway, just to err on the safe side. Clearly, this was not what I wanted to hear. However, I was somewhat reassured by the doctor's lack of concern that there wasn't something more serious afoot. At this point, the only thing I knew for sure was that I did *not* have Lyme disease.

So, Dr. Dilorenzo gave me the name of a neurologist he wanted me to see who was located in Syosset, Long Island relatively close to both my home and a short distance away from his office. He did tell me though that this doctor, Dr. Jill Bressler, did not have Saturday or evening hours and that I'd have to make an appointment to see her on a weekday. "Fine," I thought to myself, "this is great. Just what I wanted to do - take another day off from work to see a doctor." As soon as I hung up the telephone with Dr. Dilorenzo, I called Luisa and told her what he had just said. She listened and said something like, "Okay, you've got to do what you've got to do. Call this neurologist today and make an appointment." I told her I would, hung up the telephone and went back to work. I got so wrapped up with work that I forgot all about calling. Clearly, I was busy at work and was probably paying for taking a day off the prior week for my annual physical. When I got home later that evening, boy was I "scolded" for not making the appointment. Luisa and I squabbled back and forth, and I told her I would call the next morning. First thing the following day, I called Dr. Bressler's office and scheduled an appointment to see her. Thank goodness this was before Luisa called me at work later on that next morning to remind me to call the doctor to make an appointment.

Italy never looked so good!

Chapter 4
All Those Tests

After Dr. Dilorenzo referred me to a specialist, I made an appointment to see Dr. Jill Bressler, the neurologist that he used (I assumed) to see patients with unexplained neurological type symptoms. Dr. Bressler's office was located less than ten minutes from my home. I remember making an appointment to see her right after New Year's in January 2006, and going into work late one day since she only had office hours during the week.

My initial visit with Dr. Bressler was just a routine meet and greet, with a preliminary examination that lasted all of twenty minutes, if that. I probably spent more time completing the paperwork than I did seeing the doctor. After I filled out a number of new patient forms and completed some questionnaires (and of course, presenting my health insurance identification card), I was called-in from the waiting room to see Dr. Bressler; she listened to my story, asked me some questions and then did a short assessment of my strength and balance. I remember her exerting downward pressure on my arms and legs as I pushed up. She then asked me to hop on one leg with alternating feet, standing upright and in a still position – first with my eyes closed, next following her fingers with my eyes as she slowly moved them back and forth across the front of my face, and then her slightly taping/pushing me from side to side as I stood completely upright with both eyes closed. She wrote down some notes and after she was finished, she sensed my angst and gave me mild assurances that it was probably nothing to be concerned about. "You're a strong guy," I remember her saying. She did, however, order a battery of additional tests nonetheless just to be sure. She reiterated: "These tests are purely routine and I'm sure there is nothing to worry about." Like the blood test Dr. Dilorenzo ordered for Lyme disease that came-up negative, I assumed that these tests would also show nothing and that I would be fine. I thanked Dr. Bressler for her time and on my way out of the office, I scheduled the tests she had ordered. Luckily, all of the tests (except for one, the Magnetic Resonance Imaging, or MRI) could be done in the same building that her office was in. By 11 A.M., I was done with my initial appointment and was on my way headed back to work at Credit Suisse in Manhattan via the Long Island Rail Road. I completely put the visit out of my mind, not giving it any further thought until approximately two weeks later when I was scheduled to take the follow-up tests she had ordered.

I was lucky enough to be able to schedule all the tests, including the MRI, on the same day. Knowing it was going to be a long day, I remember taking off the entire day one Friday to undergo the testing. Luckily, I had enough flexibility with my job to take the entire day off (or go to work late, as necessary) so I could tend to these doctor's visits and testing appointments. I thought to myself, "What a hassle, I can't wait for this to be over." Nearly ten years later, I still have these same thoughts.

My first appointment for one of the procedures ordered by Dr. Bressler was at 8:30 A.M. at a nearby Zwanger Pesiri imaging facility that did MRI testing. I had never gone for an MRI before, so I was a bit nervous and did not know what to expect. After filling out a series of forms (and yet again having to present my health insurance identification card), I was escorted to a back "staging" room. Once there, I remember being asked to remove my watch, remove any metal jewelry I was wearing and place these and the contents of my pockets into a locker outside the MRI examination room. As I headed into the room, there were signs posted on the entrance doorway that said things in large bold letters like "Authorized Personnel Only," "No Metal Objects Permitted Beyond this Point," and "Danger – Radiation." Needless to say, the "Danger – Radiation" sign was not at all comforting!

As I entered the testing room, the technician (a young and very attractive woman, probably in her late thirties who was very amiable) asked me to lay flat on my back, face up on a long and narrow table/stretcher. She knew that I was a bit nervous, as I told her that this was the first MRI I had ever taken. Not a bad run for forty-seven years! She explained the entire process to me: I would be receiving an MRI of the brain and of the cervical spine, that it would not hurt at all but that I needed to lie perfectly still throughout the entire procedure. The long, flat, narrow stretcher I was now laying on would soon be rolled into the machine, head first, about half way up to my waist. She indicated that I would hear some very loud, banging and clanging noises throughout the procedure. Both tests, assuming I remained perfectly still, would take about forty-five minutes in total. I was told however, that if I moved, the tests would need to be started over. This was incentive enough for me to be completely obedient. I remember the room being cold and sterile looking, and the thought of having to lie on my back completely still on the long narrow "table" for another forty-five minutes would be somewhat uncomfortable. Plus, I had an appointment at Dr. Bressler's office later that morning at 11 A.M. for the next series of tests. So, I was committed to obeying the technician's instructions and not moving throughout the entire procedure. The only nice feature about the examination room, aside from it being very clean and uncluttered, was the large skylight which was positioned in the center of the ceiling. It was a very bright sunny day, so the natural sunlight which entered the room had a soothing effect on me. It also helped in somewhat warming the cold exam room.

Then, the technician asked me what kind of music I preferred. This seemed like a very odd question; would she next be asking for my phone number, my favorite restaurants? The female technician quickly went on to say that during the test, headphones would be placed over my ears to help drown out some of the noises associated with the exam, hence her question about my music preference. "Classic rock," I quickly replied!

As the stretcher I laid on was slowly rolled halfway into the machine, a set of classic rock songs played on the headphones that cupped my ears. The set of Rolling Stones, Doors and Cream songs coming through the headphones would be interrupted periodically with the technician's voice. She began by saying, "If you need anything during the test, just squeeze the button," a round rubber ball that she had placed in my right hand before the test began. Then, after the test started, her voice would occasionally interrupt the music with her saying things like: "You are doing fine" … "The next part of the exam will take about five minutes and you will hear some loud banging sounds" … "You're doing fine, just remain still"… "The next part of the test will take about ten minutes, so lie perfectly still" … "Great, how are you doing?" … "Okay, another twenty minutes, lie still" … "Don't move" … "You're doing fine" … "Almost done, home stretch now, just ten more minutes" … "Remain still. For the next few minutes you will hear some loud clanging sounds." … "You're doing fine. Don't move"… "Okay, all done."

Wow, what a relief. I was finally rolled out of the machine and able to see the sunlight through the skylight above. I'm usually not the claustrophobic type, but I was relieved to finally be out of that big, dark metal tube. As I jumped off the table (I can't do *that* anymore), I left the testing area and opened the locker outside the room and gathered my belongings. I then casually asked the technician how everything looked. (Of course, I knew full well that there was nothing she could tell me, but I asked nonetheless). As expected, I was told that I would need to consult with the prescribing physician, and that the test results would be sent to the doctor within twenty-four hours. Little did I know then that this would be the first of many MRIs to follow in the coming years. Thank goodness for headphones and classic rock!

After saying goodbye to the technician and leaving the lab, I drove the short ten mile distance to Dr. Bressler's office and was ready for the next series of tests. I got there about thirty minutes before my scheduled appointment and wound up sitting in the waiting room for just about that entire time. When I was finally called into the testing room, I remember the technician being a middle-aged gentleman who seemed as thrilled to be there as I was. There was no classic rock music that would be played this time, and no pretty young amiable female to comfort me. There was just a table in the middle of the room surrounded by some very old and large computer monitors, a set of old tattered headphones, several odd looking machines and a grumpy middle-aged male technician. At least the room I was in was comfortably heated. And oh yeah, there was no skylight in this windowless interior room.

Evoked Potential Tests (EPTs)—that was the name of the series of tests that the technician said he was instructed to administer. Nerves from different areas of my body would be tested in order to gauge my responses and the speed at which signals traveled from my brain. The test was administered in four phases in order to measure responsiveness, review electrical activity and determine reaction timing and speed.

The first in the series of tests targeted my vision and was called the Visual Evoked Potentials Test, or VEP. Here, I was asked to sit in front of a computer screen with alternating checkerboard patterns displayed, and was instructed to follow them with my eyes. The second test targeted my auditory skills and was called the Brainstem Auditory Evoked Potentials Test, or BAEP. Headphones were placed over my ears and a series of clicks were sounded in each ear. Unlike the MRI that I took previously, there were no Rolling Stones or Doors tunes played on *these* headphones; I would have much rather been listening to music though. Plus, the headphones used by the pretty MRI technician were much newer and nicer looking, and were nicely padded. In the third test, called a Sensory Evoked Potentials Test, or SEP, wires were placed on my scalp covering various parts of my head, and short electrical impulses or "shocks" were administered and transmitted to my brain. The electrical impulses, which were low voltage, did not hurt but were instead annoying. Transmission timing speeds were measured to determine the length of time it took for the electrical stimulations to travel from my brain and be felt throughout various parts of my body (mainly my arms and legs). Lastly, a Motor Evoked Potentials (MEP) test was performed in order to detect lesions along motor pathways (those that produce movement) of the central nervous system. I honestly do not remember how this test was administered, but because I was constantly asking the technician what was being done every step of the way and for what reason it was being done, I do recall that this test was performed. At this point, I was getting hungry and just wanted the tests to be done with so I could leave and grab lunch.

In all, these tests ordered by Dr. Bressler took about three hours, and were painless. Also, they must have been harmless, as there was no "Danger – Radiation" placard posted at the entranceway to the testing room. Later on, I learned that EPTs were done to measure vision proficiency and electrical activities in certain areas of the brain. I also learned that they were done in concert with other neurological lab tests to help detect potential areas of demyelination causing nerve impulses to be slowed, garbled or halted all together. I subsequently learned that EPTs were done in order to assist in the diagnosis of Multiple Sclerosis.

At the time the tests were done however, I had no clue what the doctor was testing for.

It was slightly past 3 P.M. and I was hungry, tired and ready to leave. As I departed the doctor's office and paid my co-pay to the receptionist, I asked when the test results would be available. I was told I should call by the middle of the following week, and that Dr. Bressler had office hours on Mondays, Tuesdays and Thursdays. "Okay, thank you," I said. I left, stopping quickly along the way to down a slice of pizza and put the day of testing out of my mind. When I returned home Luisa asked me how things went. My reply was very short and sweet: "Fine, what's for dinner?" I was still hungry.

I remember being at work and calling Dr. Bressler's office about 10 A.M. the following Thursday morning. "Hello, this is Vincent Spoto and I am calling to get the results of some tests I took last week." I was told by the receptionist who answered the telephone to hold a few minutes. Then, a different person came to the phone (I assume a nurse practitioner), and she told me the test results had indeed come in. I quickly asked what the results were, and was told that I needed to speak with Dr. Bressler. I remember telling the person on the other end of the telephone to let Dr. Bressler know that I was on the phone, and that she could either call me back or that I would hold until she was available to speak with me. I recall the woman on the other end of the phone saying sternly: "I'm sorry, Mr. Spoto, but Dr. Bressler will not disclose the test results to you on the telephone. She asked if you could come see her in her office. She wants to see you _today_, if possible." I immediately slouched in my chair and my heart began to race. Taking a big gulp and without thinking, I said, "Today? Sure, I guess. I am in Manhattan, but can leave my office shortly and could be there within the next couple of hours." "Okay," the nurse practitioner said. "Dr. Bressler will be in the office until 4 P.M. today, and I will let her know that you will be in to see her." I remember not uttering a word after saying goodbye and hanging-up the telephone. As I put the phone down, I slouched even lower in my chair. I was mortified!

After hanging up the telephone and feeling totally numb, my face must have turned completely ashen based on the way others on the trading floor were looking at me. My eyes welled up with tears and I was literally shaking. A few people who sat beside me on the trading desk asked if everything was okay. I remember one person, Maryann, who worked for me saying that it looked as if I had seen a ghost. She kept asking me if I was okay. She rushed and got me a cup of water. With a blank stare, I remember saying, "I'm fine, Maryann. Something has come up at home that I need to take care of." I then said that I needed to leave right away and would *not* be back to the office for the remainder of the day. Visibly shaken, I frantically called my wife and told her I was leaving the city to come home, as the doctor got the test results and wanted to see me in her office—*right away!* In a flustered voice, I told her I would pick her up on the way home from the train station before heading to the doctor's office. Frightened, I quickly hung up the phone without even giving Luisa the chance to ask any questions. I'm sure she was as shocked and as worried as I was. Like me, she was probably thinking the worst. I next quickly gathered my briefcase and bolted out of the office. I did not even put away and organize the papers on my desk. I just got up and left. On my way out, I remember popping my head into the COO's office saying I had to leave immediately, that something had come up and that I would not be back for the remainder of the day. "Family emergency," I said. "I have to leave now. I will fill you in tomorrow." I didn't even give him the chance to ask me anything.

The ten-minute walk from my office at 23rd Street and Madison Avenue to Penn Station at 34th Street and 8th Avenue to catch the Long Island Rail Road seemed like an eternity. "Brain tumor," that's all I could think it was. "A brain tumor. It must be a brain tumor." I knew I had a bad headache a few weeks back, so I thought to myself, "So of course, it has to be a brain tumor. What else could it be?"

As I boarded the train, the fifty-minute ride from Penn Station in Manhattan to the Hicksville train station in Long Island where my car was parked might as well have been fifty _hours_. I know I was in a trance, felt totally flustered and could only think of one thing: "Brain tumor. What else could it be?" I thought. "Why wouldn't the doctor come to the phone to tell me the test results?" It had to be bad. "Was I going to die? How much longer did I have left to live? Would the treatments be painful? Would I lose my hair? Would Luisa, Deanna and Lauren be okay? How would the mortgage get paid? What about paying for college? Would I be able to work ever again? How would I tell the girls? How would I tell my parents? Oh my God, what else could it be? It must be a brain tumor," I thought. "A brain tumor!"

As the train pulled into the Hicksville station and I de-boarded, I quickly walked to my car in the parking lot, got in and drove the two miles home to get Luisa. It was amazing that I was able to drive at all, as I was totally numb and glassy eyed. Red light, yellow light, green light—they all looked the same. It was remarkable I did not plow into any cars in front of me, and that I did not run any red lights. It was amazing that I was able to drive home at all! To say that I was shaken and numb is an understatement. I was in a trance. "Brain tumor. It must be a brain tumor." That's all I could think. "Brain tumor." I was very concerned, and upset, and was anxious to see the doctor. I silently prayed that she would allay my worst fears.

Luisa was anxiously waiting for me in the driveway as I pulled up to the house. She asked if I wanted her to drive. Without hesitation, I said, "Yes," and got out of the car and walked around it and sat in the passenger's seat. As she drove the short distance to the doctor's office, no words were exchanged. Blank stares permeated throughout the car ride. We were both visibly upset. On the ride over from our house to the doctor's office, there was complete silence. Neither of us even reached over to turn the car radio on. This was very atypical. We pulled into the lot of the doctor's office, parked the car and slowly walked into the building. There was no conversation. As we entered the reception area and introduced ourselves, we were told that the doctor was expecting us and to please take a seat in the waiting room. "The doctor is finishing with a patient and will be available to see you in about ten minutes," the receptionist said in a calm voice. Wow, that was the longest ten minutes ever. My heart was pounding and the silence between Luisa and I was deafening. I was holding and pretended to be reading a Highlights magazine. I was just pretending. It's hard to read when you are in a trance. How could I read anything? Then, we were called by the receptionist and escorted into Dr. Bressler's office. This was it. I had only one thing on my mind. *Brain tumor.* What else could it be?

We were asked to be seated in the two large wing chairs situated diagonally across in front of the desk in the doctor's office. Within a matter of minutes, Dr. Bressler came into the room and closed the door behind her. A middle-aged woman who was slight is stature, I remember standing and shaking Dr. Bressler's hand, and introducing her to my wife. They exchanged pleasantries. Dr. Bressler looked at the both of us stoically and said, "Okay, let's get right down to business." Luisa and I sat down on the edge of our seats. The doctor then sat down behind her desk and her demeanor was matter-of-fact; she was strictly all business. "Well, I guess you are wondering why I asked you to come in. I'll cut right to the chase. You see, I got the results from the MRI and the various other tests that you took last week. I have good news, and I have bad news," she said.

"Brain tumor," that's all I could think of.

Without any hesitation I replied, "Give me the good news first." After all, I needed something to cheer me up and get me out of the funk I was in. Without hesitation, Dr. Bressler said, "Well, it is not a brain tumor"; boy was I relieved. It was as if she could read my mind. All that worrying for nothing, so I thought. She then went on to than say that "the other piece of good news is that it is not ALS (Amyotrophic Lateral Sclerosis), also commonly known as Lou Gehrig's disease." My God, I thought, I wasn't even thinking it could be that. "That's the extent of the good news," she said.

I thought to myself - "What else could it be?"

I paused, took a deep breath and reluctantly said, "Okay, give me the bad news then." Dr. Bressler didn't hesitate, and told me that while the tests that had come back are only about 90 percent conclusive, "The MRI of the brain shows a number of white matter lesions in a pattern most suspicious of a demyelinating disease. The MRI of the cervical spine revealed an increase in signals also consistent with that of a demyelinating disease. In addition, one of the Sensory Evoked Potential Tests, or SEPs, showed response timings outside of the normal range for electric stimulations made that travel from your brain to one of your lower limbs. This, along with the MRI test results, gives me a 90 percent confidence level that you may have Multiple Sclerosis."

I paused for a brief moment. I then quickly snapped back, saying, "In English, please." Dr. Bressler's face was stoic and her response was somewhat monotone: "I cannot be 100 percent certain, but the MRI test results and those of the SEP are consistent with a diagnosis of Multiple Sclerosis." I immediately thought of Jerry's kids, and Muscular Dystrophy. I had no clue of what Multiple Sclerosis was, and asked her to explain it. "The Jerry Lewis telethon disease?" I asked. Dr. Bressler chuckled and said, "No, it has nothing to do with Muscular Dystrophy."

Believe it or not, I was somewhat relieved. After all, I did not have a brain tumor, did not have Lou Gehrig's disease (heaven forbid), and I did not have that dystrophy thing Jerry Lewis raised money for each Labor Day weekend. I also had no idea of what Multiple Sclerosis was. And, since I had never even heard of it, I figured that it couldn't be all that bad. Boy, was I mistaken! Plus, other than an occasional clumsy stumble and my legs feeling tired after long rounds of doing yardwork, I felt perfectly fine.

"Then, what is Multiple Sclerosis?", I asked. I was told by Dr. Bressler in very simple and easy to understand terms that Multiple Sclerosis is "an auto immune disease in which the disease fighting white blood corpuscles mistakenly take the myelin or insulation surrounding the nerve fibers, as bad guys." Dr. Bressler went on to say that MS occurs when the body's immune system targets its own central nervous system, i.e. the brain, spinal cord and optic nerves. When MS attacks the central nervous system, the fatty substance that protects the nerve fibers, called myelin, is damaged along with the nerve fibers themselves possibly becoming damaged. She said that after sustaining damage, the myelin forms scar tissue, in a process known as sclerosis.

I asked—"Can you put it into more simplistic language please?" Dr. Bressler did …. "Picture a wire wrapped in insulation, and the insulation that covers the wire being frayed, cracked or broken. In Multiple Sclerosis, the insulation around the wires that carry signals from your brain to various parts of your body is damaged, so the signals do not travel as quickly as they should, or may not even travel to their final destination at all. On MRIs, these damaged areas appear as lesions or spots." (Funny, to this day I use this frayed wire analogy to explain to others what Multiple Sclerosis is).

Dr. Bressler then went on to say the she was more of a general neurologist and that I may wish to consider seeing another doctor that specializes in Multiple Sclerosis. She went on to indicate that "such specialists can more carefully evaluate your case, and may order additional tests to confirm or rule-out a diagnosis of MS." For about the next minute, I just stared into her eyes, sat silently and listened. Then, Luisa and I asked a few general questions, the obvious one of course being "Will this kill me or shorten my life expectancy?" I was told emphatically that it certainly would not. "Would I wind up in a wheelchair?" I asked. "That question is premature," she said. "Everyone with Multiple Sclerosis is affected differently. And besides, I am not even 100 percent certain that you have MS." We also asked if there was an MS Specialist that she could recommend I see; Dr. Bressler did not offer a recommendation.

Still somewhat numb and bothered, we stayed at her office for a while and probably asked Dr. Bressler a bunch of questions about information that she most likely already covered. I accepted her offer for a cup of water, which she asked her assistant to bring to me. We stayed in her office for about ten more minutes and asked a few more questions. We then got up, shook Dr. Bressler's hand, thanked her for her time and left her office. Granted, we were less bothered than we were coming in, and were somewhat relieved of what my diagnosis was _not_. However, we had no clue of what Multiple Sclerosis was, so our relief was only temporary until we researched the disease on the internet at home and found out more. We pulled out of the parking lot, and I never saw Dr. Bressler again.

On the short drive home, Luisa and I were somewhat relieved - more with what the doctor said I _did not_ have as opposed to what she said I probably _did_ have. We really did not know anything about MS, so we did not realize the true meaning and extent of the condition I may have. One thing we were thankful for was that it was not something more serious, like a brain tumor or ALS. Unfortunately though, this lack of knowledge about MS was short-lived. In the weeks that followed, the more that I learned about the disease from researching it online, reading a few books on the subject that I borrowed from the library and doing some further probing, the more quickly I came to the realization that this MS thing was _NOT_ good! _Not good at all!_

Chapter 5

Seeking a Second and Third Opinion

After seeing Dr. Bressler and hearing what she said, I really did not comprehend the magnitude of what she told me, the true meaning of what Multiple Sclerosis was and the exact implications of the condition and what it meant. I didn't really know anything about MS nor did I know anyone who had it, other than a few movie and television personalities like Annette Funicello, Richard Pryor and Squiggy from *Laverne and Shirley*. In the week or two that followed in which I received the preliminary news that I might have MS, I searched the internet day and night and took out a few books from the library that discussed the disease. Within two weeks, I knew considerably more about MS than I did before, and quite frankly, more than I cared to know. What I learned was that Multiple Sclerosis is a disease of the central nervous system that affects approximately 450,000 people in the United States alone. Confirming what Dr. Bressler said, MS is believed to occur when the body's immune system attacks the fatty tissues that form sheaths (myelin) around nerve fibers within the central nervous system. The body's central nervous system, which is comprised of the brain, spinal cord and optic nerves, become scarred when the protective fatty sheaths, or myelin, become broken down. This scarring causes interruptions in the signals sent back and forth between the brain and other parts of the body. The more scaring, the more problems the body has sending and receiving signals from the brain. (This is a bit more sophisticated than the frayed wire analogy that Dr. Bressler used when first explaining the disease to me in response to my request to her for a more simplistic account of what MS is). As a result, people with MS can experience a wide range of problems including, but not limited to fatigue, muscle spasms, loss of balance and difficulty moving. Cognitive issues and mood swings represent other potential problems caused by MS.

I was no neurosurgeon, but I learned a lot about MS in a short period of time. I also read that MS patients needed to "keep moving and exercising regularly." Around this point in time, I immediately joined a gym. My joining really did not have a lot to do with anything Dr. Bressler said or recommended, and was probably largely the result of something that I wanted to do for a while anyway and had been putting off for a year or so. So I guess given what was going on with me, this seemed to be as good a time as any to join. Let's just say that my preliminary diagnosis from Dr. Bressler pushed me over the edge. And besides, even if I did not have MS, joining a gym and exercising regularly was certainly a good thing to do.

I quickly learned that MS is an autoimmune disease which manifested itself in a few different varieties. At this point though, I did not personally know anyone other than me that had MS, nor did I have any idea what type of MS I had. The only thing I was absolutely certain about was that having MS was not a good thing, and that Dr. Bressler only said that I *may* have it, but she was *not* 100 percent certain. So, my denial at this point was in full throttle and I was determined to see a neurologist who specialized in MS to get another opinion. At that present time, I had no outward everyday symptoms of the disease. And besides, the ninety percent estimate that Dr. Bressler gave me meant that there was a ten percent chance that I did not have MS. Call me the eternal optimist! Also, she ruled out my having a brain tumor as well as my having ALS. What a relief—boy, was that a huge relief! So, I researched top doctors on Long Island to determine whom I should see to get to the bottom of what was wrong with me. Finally, I came across one that piqued my interest.

Malcom Gottesman was Chief of Neurology and the Director of MS Treatment Programs at Winthrop University Hospital. I did quite a bit of research and spoke to a number of people who indicated that, in addition to being a top neurologist specializing in Multiple Sclerosis, Dr. Gottesman was extremely well regarded and a good listener who was very easy to talk with. He was also described as being very patient and selfless, and would spend the necessary time explaining things to his patients and answering their specific questions. All of the reviews I read online about him were extremely positive. Perfect, I thought to myself. I found a top neurologist that specializes in MS, a doctor who was close by, someone who could evaluate my situation and a professional who would be willing to speak with me and answer all of my questions. Such doctors, as my parents used to say, had good "bedside manners."

The earliest that I could get an appointment to see Dr. Gottesman was in the middle of March 2006. I scheduled the last possible appointment on a Thursday afternoon during the third week of March. I wanted to be certain I could make the latest appointment available so that I could leave the office as late in the day as possible so as not to miss an entire day of work. In the six weeks or so leading up to my appointment with Dr. Gottesman, I did more research online. I must have googled MS what seemed like a thousand times and I became even more knowledgeable and familiar with the disease, its different types and the treatment options available (which in the year 2006, amounted to less than a handful, with all requiring self-injection). The bad thing is that I put a lot of terrible things in my mind, and was able to confirm my initial belief that MS was not a good thing. The good news was that I was well prepared for my appointment with Dr. Gottesman. I even wrote down a whole series of questions to ask and discuss with him. And oh yeah, since I had no visible signs of the disease I was adamant that I did not have it. I guess I was in denial. True, there were some days when I would come home from work around 8 P.M. (which was the norm), and be beat. But most days I felt perfectly fine. I attributed my occasional fatigue to awakening at 5:30 A.M. each morning, putting in a ten to twelve hour day, dealing with some very stressful situations at work, getting home some days after 8 P.M. and just getting older. But that was it; everything else seemed fine. Still, I was resolute in my belief that I did not have MS and that my relatively infrequent stumbles were just due to pure clumsiness, my overall lack of coordination, the result of some obscure virus that could quickly be treated and cured or something that simply would go away on its own.

I remember my first appointment with Dr. Gottesman. I took the Long Island Rail Road train from Manhattan directly to his office across from Winthrop University Hospital in Mineola. I was well prepared. I had all my questions written down and well organized, and came with a folder containing copies of the test results taken as a result of my previous visits with Dr. Bressler. I also brought with me a CD Rom that had a picture of my brain and spine from the MRI I had taken in January that was used to preliminarily diagnose my condition. Luisa, who met me at Dr. Gottesman's office, had all her questions in her mind. Unlike me, she was able to rattle them off from memory and did not have to write things down or prepare any notes. This was consistent with the approach she took on most things, and was not a surprise.

After filling out a series of new patient forms which took nearly twenty minutes to complete, I handed the papers to the receptionist along with a folder containing my prior test results and the CD Rom with images of my MRI. The receptionist took all of my documents and the completed papers, and almost immediately asked for my health insurance card, which she photocopied and returned. (I quickly was beginning to realize that without a card evidencing that you have health insurance, you literally have to go to the back of the line—that is if you are allowed to get on the line at all)! I could only imagine what would have happened if I said I did not have my insurance card with me; I'm sure I would have been politely told to "scram" and come back at a later date when I had it. But since I was able to provide the card when asked, miraculously (after another ten minutes passed) a nurse practitioner came out to the waiting room to greet Luisa and I and escort us to an examination room. She walked us down a hallway to a corner room and said to be seated, make ourselves comfortable and that Dr. Gottesman would be in to see [us] shortly after he had completed reviewing the prior test results that we provided. So, we sat and waited. After about ten minutes, the doctor came into the room.

Dr. Gottesman was a rather unassuming and distinguished looking man, not very tall, with graying hair and in his mid fifties (if I had to guess). He had a soft but firm voice and appeared very friendly. As he listened attentively and peered at me over spectacles that rested on the bridge of his nose, I told him the history of what brought me in to see him. As I took him through my story, Dr. Gottesman immediately made Luisa and I feel very comfortable. Quickly, I came to the conclusion that what I had heard about Dr. Gottesman being a good listener who was very easy to talk with was entirely accurate. I liked him and felt at ease, as I responded to a series of questions he asked throughout my preliminary examination. He appeared to be very knowledgeable about MS, and at times throughout the discussion Luisa would interject and add certain things she had noticed from watching me in the past. She would also ask an occasional question. Dr. Gottesman listened attentively, asked follow-up questions and acknowledged that Luisa had some critical insights she garnered from watching me that were important and needed to be considered. I sat quietly and observed the interchange.

After he and Luisa finished their exchange, Dr. Gottesman next did a quick assessment of my strength and balance (similar to the assessment done during my previous visit with Dr. Bressler). When he was finished, Dr. Gottesman directed our attention to a computer screen which showed the CD Rom images of my brain and of my spine that were taken from my MRIs. He also had a second computer screen in the room showing the MRI image of a normal brain and spine. This allowed him to very easily illustrate to me the differences between the two sets of images. While very interesting, I wasn't exactly sure what I was looking at. However, I assumed that there were differences in the images appearing on the two screens. I guess the saying that "a picture is worth a thousand words" is true. Dr. Gottesman pointed out several areas on my MRI screen which he said appeared to show some lesions consistent with those found in patients having Multiple Sclerosis. He was quick to say however, that the appearance of these spots was not conclusive evidence that I did have MS. He also pointed out that there was some slight atrophy of my brain which he said was consistent with an individual in my age group, and that it may or may not necessarily have anything to do with a potential diagnosis of MS.

Next, Dr. Gottesman took us through his review of my EPT test results. He explained that only one of the four tests, the Sensory Evoked Potentials Test (or SEP), showed some things that were outside of the normal range. Specifically, he noted that response times to electric stimulations made on my scalp and transmitted from my brain to various parts of my limbs were slower than normal. He then told us that the tests that were taken to date, both the MRIs and the SEPs, were still inconclusive at this point regarding a 100 percent positive diagnosis of MS. He said that he would like me to re-take two additional MRIs, one of the brain and the other of the cervical spine, both with and without contrast (referred to as gadolinium). I learned later that gadolinium was a liquid injected into one's veins when taking an MRI in order to enhance images and assist in a more accurate diagnosis. At this point, Dr. Gottesman concluded the initial consultation and wrote two scripts for the MRIs. He said that a few days after I took the MRIs I should schedule another appointment to see him in order to review the results. We shook hands with him, said goodbye and left his office. All in all, my initial visit with Dr. Gottesman ran about forty minutes. Dr. Gottesman—what a nice man!

Approximately two weeks later, I was back at Zwanger Pesiri to take the two MRIs that were ordered by Dr. Gottesman. This time, there was no paperwork to fill out (since this was my second visit to the lab within the past sixty days); I was a seasoned veteran. Unlike the previous MRIs, there was a point where a dye called gadolinium was injected into my veins prior to testing. This time the technician was a middle aged male who joked as he injected the dye into my arm and said something like, "This is so your insides will light up like a pinball machine." After the injection, I knew the routine. All metal objects, jewelry and my watch had to be removed and placed in a locker outside of the testing room before entering. As I entered the imaging room (the same one by the way that I had used previously), I glanced over at the posted sign that said "Danger - Radiation." Once inside the room, I laid face-up on a long narrow table, donned a set of headphones playing classic rock music and was rolled into the MRI imaging machine up to my waste. This time, instead of taking forty-five minutes, I remained on the table inside the testing room for about one hour. And for this hour, I endured loud clanging and banging sounds like I did with the MRI that I had taken previously. Only this time there were fewer interruptions from the technician's voice. The music was good though! The exam room was still quite cool and sterile looking. It was a cloudy day so the skylight above really did little to brighten things up inside the room.

After about one hour, the technician said, "All done." I jumped off the table, went outside of the imaging room to my locker, gathered my belongings and left. It was about 10:30 A.M. and I headed to the Hicksville train station to catch the Long Island Rail Road into Manhattan. My goal was to get into the office by noon. I made it.

About two weeks later in mid-April 2006, I made an appointment to see Dr. Gottesman in order to review the test results. Like I did previously, I made the appointment as late in the day as possible in order to minimize my time away from the office. This time, I flew solo as Luisa was unable to come with me. I remember sitting in the waiting room for about twenty minutes before being called in to see Dr. Gottesman. While sitting there, I struck-up a conversation with a middle-aged man sitting across from me in a wheelchair. An ex-New York City police officer, we began talking and he (I'll refer to him as Bill) told me that he had been a patient of Dr. Gottesman's for a number of years and that he suffered from Multiple Sclerosis. Bill appeared to be in his forties and said that because of his condition, he was forced to quit the police force and retire with full disability several years ago. I listened attentively, smiling and nodding as he spoke. I was careful not to ask too many questions but really didn't need to, as Bill spoke openly and freely about his condition. He did not hesitate to share information with me about his life and his situation. At times, I thought he gave out too much information; stuff I didn't really need (or want) to know. But, I listened anyway. Bill felt like talking.

He told me that he was diagnosed with MS in 1996 after he began experiencing double vision and tingling sensations both in his arms and legs. Within a few years he said he was unable to walk freely, required the assistance of a walker and needed to quit his job with the police force and go onto permanent disability. Shortly thereafter, he began utilizing a motorized scooter. This was not a story I wanted to hear, albeit I politely listened and smiled nonetheless. Bill went on to talk about

Dr. Gottesman, saying what a wonderful neurologist he is and how he put him on the drug Copaxone (which he remained on currently) shortly after he was diagnosed. He praised Dr. Gottesman and said that he was the only neurologist he ever used to treat his MS. At that point, I was called by the receptionist and told that Dr. Gottesman was ready to see me. I stood, shook Bill's hand and wished him the best for the future. He gave me his best wishes as well and wished me good luck. Several years later I remember briefly "running" into Bill at a restaurant where an MS information session was being held that discussed various treatment options. Bill was still utilizing a motorized scooter, and looked pretty much the same.

As I left the waiting area, I was escorted to an examination room by one of the office assistants and asked to be seated. I was told that Dr. Gottesman would be in to see me shortly and sure enough within five minutes, Dr. Gottesman came into the room and sat across from me. We exchanged pleasantries, and then he began saying that he had an opportunity to review my test results and compare them to the ones taken previously as ordered by Dr. Bressler. He said that the MRIs of both the cervical spine and brain showed multiple areas of signal abnormality with an appearance strongly suggestive of an inflammatory demyelinating disorder. He went on to tell me that while several lesions were identified, none of them demonstrated any contrast enhancement. (I wasn't quite certain what that meant, but it sure sounded like a good thing). While not 100 percent certain, Dr. Gottesman said that the test results suggested to him that the demyelinating disorder may in fact be Multiple Sclerosis. I paused, and then asked. "How do we find out for sure?"

Dr. Gottesman indicated that the only real way to be certain, or at least be as close to 100 percent positive as possible, would be to extract and analyze fluid taken from my spinal cord. A lumbar puncture, or spinal tap, was what he recommended. Oh boy, this did _not_ have a good sound to it. I went onto to ask Dr. Gottesman about the procedure. He proceeded to tell me that is something he himself does and that it was a one half day out-patient procedure that needed to be done in the hospital. He went on to tell me that he generally did the procedure in the morning, it took about an hour or two and that it did not require the use of anesthesia. I asked about side-effects. Other than feeling some slight discomfort throughout the procedure, he indicated that some of his patients experienced a strong headache for the remainder of the day, with a very small number of patients experiencing nausea either during or shortly after the procedure. As such, he recommends to his patients that undergo a spinal tap to take the entire day off from work and not do anything for twenty-four hours or so that might involve strenuous or rapid movement. Other than a headache and the remote possibility of feeling nauseous, he indicated that a small number of his patients who underwent the procedure said it was somewhat uncomfortable. "Great," I thought to myself. "Just what I wanted to hear, another test (which in this case may be uncomfortable may make me nauseous), and another need to take a day off from work."

I told Dr. Gottesman that I probably would go forward with the procedure, but that I wanted first to discuss it with my wife and that I would then call to let him know for certain. He seemed very compassionate, said he understood and that he would wait for my call. I shook his hand and thanked him (for what, I don't know), then drove home. I was concerned and somewhat confused. When I got home, I explained to Luisa what Dr. Gottesman said. Without hesitation she said I should undergo the procedure. We talked for a bit afterwards, and I then called Dr. Gottesman's office later that day to advise him of my decision to proceed. I spoke to his receptionist who indicated that Dr. Gottesman was gone for the day but that she would relay my message to him in the morning. In the meantime she said she would proceed with obtaining the necessary approvals from my health insurance provider. Once approved, she would be in contact with me to set-up an appointment for the procedure.

By this point both Luisa and I had a strong suspicion that I might have MS. We didn't really say anything, as we usually avoided the topic and tried to put the possibility of my having MS out of our minds. At times, it was awkward not talking about the subject and ignoring it. But, I had the feeling that MS may very well be in the card-hand which I was dealt. I was never a great poker player but this time, as fate would have it and would later be determined, I had a "full house"!

About two weeks later toward the end of May, everything was set for the lumbar puncture (aka spinal tap). I made an appointment for early one Friday morning at Winthrop University Hospital with Dr. Gottesman to undergo the procedure. And yes, I had to take another full day off from work. Luisa accompanied me to the hospital. I purposely scheduled the procedure for a Friday so that I would not have to worry about going into work the next day in case any issues arose later on that day or the next. To say I was nervous in the days leading-up to the procedure was an understatement. I am generally not one to worry, but sleeping the night before was not easy. I tossed and turned and would awaken periodically thinking about and dreading what lied ahead. The thought of having a long, cold needle inserted into my spine was not at all comforting and certainly was not conducive to having a restful and uninterrupted sleep.

The next day, Dr. Gottesman greeted Luisa and I at the hospital and accompanied us to the room where the spinal tap was to be performed. Prior to that, I remember completing and signing a number of information disclosures and authorization forms in the out-patient admitting area. And of course, I had to once again show my healthcare insurance identification card. Luisa went into the examination room with me. The spinal tap itself was relatively painless, and a surprisingly quick procedure. I remember it taking all of about forty-five minutes and yes, it was a bit uncomfortable but not really all that painful. Preparation of the site (i.e. disinfecting the area with alcohol swabs, numbing the area on my lower back, preparing the needle and the vial to extract and store the fluid, etc.) probably took as much time as the actual procedure itself did. The high level of anxiety that built-up inside of me leading up to the spinal tap was a lot worse than the actual procedure itself was. Every step of the way, Dr. Gottesman talked me through the process. He could not have been more comforting and re-assuring. Dr. Gottesman even took the time to show me the needle he would be inserting into my back to extract the spinal fluid. This was not really something that I wanted to see, but he explained that it was important for me to be familiar with every aspect of the procedure so that I was totally aware of the process.

Even though he numbed the area I remember feeling a slight pinch as he inserted the needle into my spine, and it being somewhat uncomfortable for the minute or so that the needle was inside of me and the fluid was being extracted. Before I knew it, he was uttering the words I wanted to hear: "All done." Wow, I thought! This procedure, while not something I would recommend to others, was not as bad as I thought it would be. Granted, I was still unsure of what discomforts may lay ahead for the remainder of the day and the upcoming weekend. After the spinal-tap was done, Dr. Gottesman told me to call him later on that day to let him know how I was doing. He told me to take two Tylenol every four hours for the remainder of the day, and to be sure not do anything strenuous and to just sit on the couch, rest and watch television. He repeated himself sternly saying, "No lifting or strenuous activities." He also said I should call him on Tuesday of the following week to schedule an appointment to review and discuss the results. I called his office later that day and left a message with his nurse assistant that I was doing fine. The remainder of the weekend was relatively uneventful, and I went back to work in the city the following Monday as normal. Everyone I spoke with previously was right about Dr. Gottesman's demeanor and his overall approach to things. He really did have excellent "bedside manners."

The next week I called Dr. Gottesman's office to get the results of the spinal tap. He came to the phone and indicated that the results came back positive and that I likely *did* have MS. My worst fear had been confirmed! He was direct and somewhat matter-of-fact. I paused for a bit, and then asked him in a low solemn voice what the next steps should be. By this point, I was somewhat resigned to the fact that I had MS, albeit remotely hopeful, very remotely hopeful that this was not the case. He said I should schedule an appointment to come see him in his office to discuss next steps and potential treatment options. I said yes I would, at which point Dr. Gottesman transferred me over to his office manager in order to schedule a follow-up appointment for me to meet with him. I scheduled the appointment to see him late in the day the following Thursday afternoon.

This time, Luisa accompanied me when I went to see Dr. Gottesman at his office. He seemed almost apologetic for having to give me the news that I most likely had MS. He explained that because it was unclear as to whether or not there were any real defined instances of relapses or exacerbations, it was pretty much unknown to him the exact form of MS that I might have—relapsing remitting or progressive. He was leaning more toward the progressive form though. He also said that no two cases of MS are the same, and indicated how everyone who has MS has distinctive symptoms. He further elaborated by saying that those who have MS experience different things, ranging from having no symptoms at all, to having extreme fatigue, to having rounds of double vision, to having tingling sensations in their arms and legs, to experiencing weakness in their limbs, to having challenges with balance and walking, to experiencing bowel or bladder issues, etc. "Oh boy," I thought to myself. Dr. Gottesman went on to say that "in your case, since you currently are not showing any symptoms or experiencing any issues, it's probably okay if you take some time to think about things before you start therapy. The fact that you currently do not have any visible symptoms or are experiencing any flare-ups is a good thing."

Dr. Gottesman said that Copaxone was a medication he thought may be best for me, but he told me I should think about it and know that administering it required having to give myself a daily injection. "Copaxone," he told me, "had a high level of efficacy, has shown positive results in slowing disease progression and has relatively few minor, if any minor side-effects." I listened. The thought of giving myself daily injections frightened me. Being somewhat knowledgeable by this point in time about MS (thank goodness for Google), I knew that it was advisable to begin drug treatments early upon diagnosis in order to slow or stop progression of the disease. As such, Luisa and I both agreed to talk things over amongst ourselves but first asked Dr. Gottesman if I should start taking the medication now. Dr. Gottesman reiterated what he already said: "Think about it and let me know what you decide." Injecting myself every day was *really* not something I wanted to do. Plus, taking a drug daily was not something I would do so hastily without doing ample research.

Then it hit me: "Oh my God," I thought, "this MS thing is for real!" Visibly shaken, I told Dr. Gottesman I wasn't sure if I was ready to start treatment and begin taking daily injections. He was comforting in saying that this was not a decision that needed to be made today, especially since I had no real visible symptoms at the present time. He offered me a drink of water (which I accepted), and again said that Copaxone is the course of treatment he would likely recommend. At that point, Dr. Gottesman left the room for a few minutes to give Luisa and I some time to talk amongst ourselves.

We were both torn between the rudimentary knowledge we had about the disease which strongly stressed and highly recommended the need to begin treatment upon diagnosis, and the reality that I needed to give myself daily injections. Clearly, Dr. Gottesman was the expert and someone whose recommendation we deemed to be important and strongly worthy of considering. He was a very experienced and knowledgeable man; a caring physician who really knew his stuff. Luisa sensed that I was leaning toward getting another opinion though, and was fully supportive. With respect to Dr. Gottesman, I could not help but think of what my mom would always say when talking about factors to consider when choosing a first-rate doctor; be sure he or she has good "bedside manners." One thing was clear at this point though – Dr. Gottesman *did* have excellent "bedside manners."

When Dr. Gottesman returned to the room, I was very up front with him. I told him that I still had a lot of thinking to do, and that I would likely be seeking another opinion. He totally understood, saying that getting the news of having MS is quite traumatic and that if he were in my shoes, he would probably do the same thing and seek a second opinion. We shook hands with Dr. Gottesman, thanked him for his time and for all the assistance he provided to date and that we would let him know of our plans for proceeding. Cordial and gracious, Dr. Gottesman said that we should feel free to call him at any time should we have any questions or need any additional information in helping to make a decision. We drove home, had dinner and did not speak a lot about what we had just been told. The reality that I had MS hadn't fully "sunk in" yet, and I imagine Luisa and I were both trying to digest the news. After dinner, I immediately "hit the computer" and did some research online looking for Long Island and New York City based neurologists specializing in MS in my quest to garner a second opinion.

I spent the next few hours searching the computer about Multiple Sclerosis, existing and experimental therapies, top doctor's specializing in the field, etc. A number of names came up, including Dr. Gottesman's. I further narrowed my search to look for neurologists specializing in

MS that were well known, very experienced and had a history of being aggressive relating to pursuing and administering treatment options. Because of the "aggressive treatment options" phrase that I included in my search and the fact that I further limited it to Long Island and New York City based doctors, the results were minimal. This was what I expected. However, there was one name that came up a number of times. Specifically, this physician had a fair number of patient testimonials online speaking to her strong credentials, along with the aggressive manner in which she provided care. I guess it was a long shot, but my search for a well-known neurologist specializing in MS and known for administering aggressive treatment was a "hit."

It was Dr. Karen Blitz-Shabbir. The Director of the North Shore MS Care Center in East Meadow, Long Island and the Director of Neuro rehabilitation at North Shore University Hospital at Glen Cove. Dr. Blitz was also listed as the attending neurologist at Nassau University Medical Center in East Meadow and cited as being a well-known speaker on treatment issues concerning MS. In addition, Dr. Blitz was noted as being a member of the New York State Consortium of MS Centers, the American Academy of Neurology, and the American Society of Neuro rehabilitation. To boot, there were several patient testimonials indicating that Dr. Blitz had a "no-nonsense" demeanor about her, and that she was very direct and aggressive in treating her patients. "Great," I thought, "this is exactly what I was looking for." I jotted down the names of some of the individuals that provided the testimonials, and was determined to contact them prior to making a decision to see her.

The following week I proceeded to contact three of the individuals who had written online testimonials; two were existing patients and one was a former patient. It took a few days, but I was able to track-down contact information for each of them. I sent emails to them saying what I was inquiring about and asked if it would be okay if I were to phone them at a convenient time. All three people went out of their way to respond to my request almost immediately, with each of them getting back to me and providing me with their phone numbers along with the best times to call. Funny, because one thing I was beginning to quickly realize was that people who had MS went out of their way to talk with and assist others. To this day I still find this to be the case, and always do the same when I am approached by others with questions about the disease.

Over the next week, I phoned and spoke with all three people. Unanimously, they all praised Dr. Blitz for the deep knowledge and experience she had regarding MS. When I spoke with them about the treatments they were receiving, each of them told me that Dr. Blitz was aggressive in recommending new and different therapy options. Each of them indicated that Dr. Blitz would consistently reevaluate their progress real-time during each visit and was not afraid to propose new treatment recommendations that she deemed appropriate if warranted under the circumstances. I asked the one person who was a former patient why she left her. She said that she needed to leave and make arrangements to see another doctor for convenience reasons due to her moving from Long Island to Westchester County in New York. This person was truly not happy with having to leave Dr. Blitz and missed the doctor's vast knowledge of MS and her direct style. However, she was unable (and unwilling) to endure the ninety + minute drive from Westchester to the doctor's office in East Meadow, Long Island. I clearly understood.

In addition to each person speaking highly of Dr. Blitz's knowledge and skills, they also talked about the "matter-of-fact," "no-nonsense" approach she took with her patients. In fact one person elaborated further by saying they were aware of two people who had left Dr. Blitz for another physician, citing that they were "turned off" by her blunt, direct style and wished she would have come across "warmer." Finally, as I explained my situation to each person, they all recommended to me that Dr. Blitz was the doctor I should see. Each of them gave me their unqualified recommendations. One person went as far to say that "If I were in your shoes, I would not hesitate to see Blitz." After speaking with each person, I chatted with Luisa about the feedback I had obtained. We agreed that the goal was to see the best and most assertive doctor possible and not to necessarily see the friendliest, warmest and most amiable doctor that may not have the strongest medical background and experience in dealing with MS. After all, this was not about entering a popularity contest! Luisa and I agreed what the next steps should be.

My decision was made. It was Dr. Blitz I would see, provided she would accept me as a new patient.

Chapter 6

The Results Are In: Time to Start Treatment

The following Monday in early June I called Dr. Blitz's office and spoke with her assistant, Donna, about my situation and reason for me wanting to see her. Donna was very kind and took all my information over the telephone, and said she would speak with Dr. Blitz and get back to me. Later on that day, Donna called me back and said that Dr. Blitz, who was extremely busy, would see me but that the earliest appointment she could give me as a new patient would be mid-July (or in six weeks). I tried, but was unsuccessful at negotiating a sooner appointment. I accepted the mid-July date, and was told by Donna to bring with me all of my prior test results and scans. While I was not thrilled with having to wait so long to see her, I was at least fortunate enough that Dr. Blitz agreed to meet with me for an initial consultation.

I remember my first visit to see Dr. Blitz. It was a very hot and humid weekday toward the end of July 2006. I happened to have been starting my two week vacation that week, so there was no need to take a day off from work; Luisa accompanied me to see Dr. Blitz at her office in Glen Cove Hospital. I later learned that her primary office was located in East Meadow, Long Island, and that she was only at the Glen

Cove office one day per week. (I subsequently discovered that I was only able to schedule the appointment as soon as I did because I opted to see her in her office at Glen Cove Hospital, and that Dr. Blitz usually saw patients in her East Meadow office). From the time I became a patient of Dr. Blitz, this was my one-and-only visit to her Glen Cove office; all my future visits to see her would be in East Meadow.

As a new patient, I knew to arrive about thirty to forty-five minutes prior to my noon appointment so that I could complete the myriad of paperwork that awaited me. And of course, I was sure to bring my healthcare insurance identification card. I also brought with me copies of all the test results and scans I had accumulated since the beginning of the year. Completion of the paperwork was somewhat seamless and quick, as Donna was quite helpful in expediting the process. With all the paperwork complete, I was asked by Donna to take a seat in a small waiting area and told that it may be a while before Dr. Blitz could see us, as she was making rounds in the hospital visiting with patients. Lusia and I made ourselves comfortable flipping through numerous issues of *People* magazine and *Business Week*, and that day's edition of the *Daily News*. I also stumbled (what an operative word that would later become) upon an issue of *Neurology Today* which I found very interesting, as it had a feature article about a patient living with MS and the pain she was enduring. ("Pain," I thought to myself. "Hmm, no one ever said anything about that to me.") About forty minutes had gone by and after two interruptions from Donna offering apologies for the doctor's tardiness, Dr. Blitz was back in her office and ready to see us. We left the waiting area and were accompanied by Donna into Dr. Blitz's office around 12:45 P.M.

Karen Blitz was a professional and pensive looking middle-aged woman (in her late forties if I had to guess), about 5'6", with short dark hair and appearing to be very fit. She was impeccably dressed and seemed somewhat out of breath, presumably from making her rounds in the hospital. She warmly greeted us and apologized for keeping us waiting. An amiable individual but seemingly a "no-nonsense" type, Dr. Blitz got right down to business and asked why I was here to see her and how she could assist. I immediately liked her direct and forthright style. I began telling her my story, and handed her the folder I brought with me that contained all the test results and copies of the scans that I had taken over the past several months. I proceeded to tell my story, going all the way back to the beginning in 2005 when I first felt weaknesses in my legs when I was doing yardwork. She frequently asked me questions throughout the visit, as I took her through the events of the past eighteen months which brought me in to see her. A common theme in her inquiries centered on fatigue and if I noticed anything different relating to my stamina. I responded that I had not noticed anything out of the ordinary, other than occasionally feeling tired at the end of certain days and going to bed early as a result. I went on to tell her that I generally felt fine the following morning and was then usually back to my energetic self. She asked if in general, I noticed any difference in my energy level at the start of each day versus how I felt in the evenings or on days when I experienced the fatigue. Her probing made me reflect and ponder before answering.

"Come to think of it," I said, "on most days, I feel more energetic in the mornings than I do in the evenings, but nothing extreme." I continued, and I recall saying (I guess I'm paraphrasing, as I don't remember the exact words that I used): "It's funny because this weary and tired feeling that I experience toward the end of certain days only happens to me once in a while, like a few times a month particularly when it is very hot and humid. But when it does happen, it only lasts for a day or so and then I'm fine. Also as I think back, there were a few times over the past couple of months when I was cleaning out my car, or a closet, and one time when I was organizing the work room of my garage when I suddenly got very tired and just felt 'off,' almost like I had too much to drink." "How long did it last?" she asked. I replied, "One time the feeling lasted a few days. The other times, it went away after I sat down and rested for a short while. And like I said, most times I felt fine and as energetic as normal the next morning." Dr. Blitz nodded and had a somber look on her face, and wrote down some notes as I spoke. Luisa seemed surprised by what I was saying, as I really never mentioned anything to her about this. I guess that's because I really didn't see it as anything out of the norm, and attributed it to just getting older.

Dr. Blitz went on to ask about the type of work I did, if I had a lot of stress and about my travel schedule and frequency. Again paraphrasing, I said, "I work in a Wall Street office, investment banking. Yeah, there is a fair amount of stress, particularly with meeting deadlines imposed by senior management. I work in a fast-paced environment and dealing with traders, investors and regulators always poses a challenge. This is especially so when dealing with the traders, as they want everything 'yesterday.' Regarding travel, I'm probably on the road about twenty to twenty-five percent of the time. The good news here is that I generally choose when to go on the road and basically have full control of my travel schedule," I replied. "Do you manage people?" Dr. Blitz asked. "Yes," I responded, "but I direct professionals." I recall telling her that of course there is always some degree of stress and there are certain challenges that come about whenever supervising people, regardless of their level. I let her know that in general though, I liked what I did and enjoyed the people I worked with. "They are self-starters and require little direction," I said. Dr. Blitz went on and asked if I had noticed any changes in my cognitive abilities, i.e. memory lapses, difficulty in finding the right words when speaking or writing, etc. "No," I said, "nothing at all comes to mind on the cognitive front." Luisa laughed, and said that I always had selective memory anyway. "Be honest," Luisa said, "you frequently forget things I say and ask you to do." Dr. Blitz laughed and said that she's heard that from patient's spouses many times before. "Sure sounds like selective memory," Dr. Blitz said as she smiled and laughed. She then asked, "Nothing out of the ordinary, though, right?" Both Luisa and I almost simultaneously said, "No, nothing out of the ordinary comes to mind."

I continued telling Dr. Blitz my story and she asked questions throughout my visit. "Any pain? Any numbness or tingling sensations in your arms or legs? Have you had any double vision or have you experienced any issues with your eyesight? Have you experienced any bowel or bladder problems? Have you noticed any changes in your handwriting?" Throughout the consultation I responded that I had never experienced any pain, other than the normal aches and pains associated with aging. I also told her that I really have never experienced any numbness or tingling sensations in my arms or legs, and that I do not have any vision issues either. I indicated to her that on very rare occasions, bladder voiding seemed to take more time than usual, but that my bowel functionality has always been and continues to be fine. I then told her that my handwriting is probably as bad today as it has always been. "Let's put it this way," I said, "my handwriting has certainly _not_ gotten any better over the years." There were probably other questions that she asked throughout the exam, but these are the ones I can remember.

Next, she looked at the test results I had given her and then popped into her desktop computer the CD ROMs I had brought with me. She really did not spend much time studying the images, but instead spent the majority of her time reading through the narratives that summarized the test results while speaking directly with me. Dr. Blitz then did a short assessment of my strength, similar to the assessments done previously by both doctors Bressler and Gottesman. Dr. Blitz exerted downward pressure separately on both my arms and legs as I pushed up. She asked me to hop on my left foot, then on my right foot. When I was done hopping, I was asked to tap the ground separately with each foot, and then asked to stand upright in a still position with both of my eyes closed. After a few minutes, she asked that I open my eyes. Next, she gradually moved her fingers back and forth across the front of my face and asked me to follow them with my eyes. Then, she asked me to walk backwards and from side to side. Next she asked me to stand upright as she slightly tapped and pushed me, first on my left side and then on my right side on an alternating basis. She did this as I stood completely still with both eyes closed. I guess she was trying to see if I could maintain my balance and not be pushed over. I passed, and was determined to show her that I was no "pushover!" Throughout all of this, Dr. Blitz occasionally jotted down some notes.

At this point I had been with Dr. Blitz for approximately forty-five minutes, and I felt she was really giving me a very thorough examination. Afterwards, Luisa and I spoke and commented on how thorough we felt the initial consultation was. "Well," Dr. Blitz said, not mincing any words, "from what I can see from examining you and from what you have told me, by looking at the results from the MRIs you had done, by reviewing the results of the Evoked Potential Tests, by looking at the results of the spinal tap and by reviewing the notes written by both Dr. Bressler and Dr. Gottesman, I am 99 percent certain that you have Multiple Sclerosis." She was direct, straight forward and did not beat around the bush. My deepest fear had now become a reality—I did have MS!

I leaned back in the chair, was in total silence and I'm sure I had a blank stare on my face. I asked Dr. Blitz if she was sure. She reiterated what she had just told me: "I am 99 percent sure." I slowly began to realize that the results I had feared were true. Dr. Blitz confirmed the initial assessments and inclinations of the prior two doctors who saw me. I had MS. Both Luisa and I were somewhat in shock, even though the events which led up to my initial visit with Dr. Blitz all pointed toward the fact that I had the disease. I guess we both were in denial.

I composed myself and was slowly coming to the realization that I did in fact have MS. I glanced over at Luisa and she too looked upset. I was somewhat relieved however, that there was more or less of a consensus among a number of leading neurologists in that they knew what was wrong with me. Still though, I was dazed and upset. Lyme disease never looked so good! After spending close to one hour with Dr. Blitz, I was pretty convinced that the diagnosis was real and that the results were pretty final. I did not see any need to get another opinion.

Dr. Blitz went on to say, "I'm sure you're wondering why I say that I am 99 percent versus 100 percent sure that you have the disease. You see, MS symptoms vary from patient to patient and therefore a 100 percent conclusive diagnosis is very difficult to make." I nodded my head conveying my understanding. Next she said, "I'm sure you also want to know what type of MS you have." I again nodded, slowly moving my head up and down. "Relapsing Remitting MS (RRMS) is what I believe you have." Somewhat surprised, I told her that my understanding was that RRMS was characterized by specific attacks and relapses and that I really had not experienced any, at least any that I could recall. After all, I was now an MS expert, being a recent graduate of "Google University."

"I disagree," she said. "The heaviness you felt in your legs when doing yardwork, the fatigue you experienced toward the end of some days that sometimes lingered on for a few days, your intolerance to heat, the tired and 'off' feeling that you mentioned when performing certain tasks around the house, the occasional bladder voiding issues you've experienced—I consider each one of these to be exacerbations. Granted, while these may seem mild and do not appear to be significant, I still consider them to be exacerbations." After I paused, I took a deep breath and nodded. I asked her about next steps and the timing as to if and when I should start treatment. Without even the blink of an eye, she instantly responded, "You need to start treatment immediately!" Wow, the patient testimonials I had read about Dr. Blitz were true. She did not mince words, was quite direct and was very aggressive in recommending that I start immediate treatment.

Almost instantaneously I asked, "Copaxone?" Dr. Blitz responded by saying, "No, I would like to put you on Avonex. Like Copaxone, Avonex must be administered via injection. But unlike Copoxone where injections are done daily, Avonex is injected [by the patient] weekly." (Hmmm, weekly versus a daily injection—that sounded a lot better). I asked about the difference between the two drugs and she pointed out that Avonex, unlike Copaxone, is in a class of drugs called interferons and that she was more comfortable in my case recommending this as an initial treatment option. Dr. Blitz went on to also tell me that unlike Copaxone which is injected subcutaneously (in the fat layer between the skin and the muscle), Avonex is injected directly into the muscle (intramuscularly). I would later research all of the various MS drugs on the market at that time and become more knowledgeable about how they worked, how they were administered, their side-effects, their effectiveness, etc. And I quickly learned that intramuscular injections, like those done for Avonex, were administered directly into the muscle using a longer needle. YIKES!

I asked Dr. Blitz about the side-effects associated with Avonex and she told me that all drugs have side-effects to some degree. She then said that "with Avonex, we just need to monitor your blood once per quarter to be sure there are no adverse effects on your liver. Also Avonex, like all interferons, sometimes causes flu like symptoms in patients, especially early on when they are first used. I recommend that my patients on Avonex take two Aspirin or Tylenol prior to giving themselves the injection, and then take another two pills before going to bed that evening." I kept telling myself that if there was any *good news* it was that Avonex was administered weekly, unlike Copaxone which needed to be administered every day. The *bad news* was that I had to give myself a weekly injection directly into the muscle, using of course a longer needle. And of course, *ultimately the "bad news"* was that I had been diagnosed with MS.

At the conclusion of my initial visit with Dr. Blitz, I gave her my consent to move ahead and contact my insurance company so that the necessary approvals could be obtained so that the drug could be ordered and I could begin treatment. She told me that "once the approval from your insurance company is obtained, Donna will be contacting you to let you know so you can order the medicine. At that time, Donna will be scheduling an appointment for you in the East Meadow office so that our Nurse Practitioner Mary Jean Buhse can spend time 'training' you on how to give yourself the injections." Both Luisa and I stood and shook hands with Dr. Blitz and thanked her for the time she spent with us. It was now around 2 P.M., and we said goodbye to her and left. My initial impression: Dr. Blitz knew her stuff and did not waste any time getting down to business. I liked that!

Two days later, Donna called to tell me that the necessary approvals were obtained from my medical insurance carrier and I could proceed with calling the pharmacy to order the drug (uugghhh, I couldn't wait!). Avonex came in a thirty day supply and was dispensed via mail order only. Donna then asked for my availability to schedule a follow-up appointment for "training" on how to administer the drug. Since I was also going to be on my second week of vacation the following week, I asked and was successful in scheduling an appointment for the following Thursday. "Be sure you allocate about one hour for this visit so that Mary Jean can show you how to do the injections," Donna said. I thanked her and hung up. I immediately placed a call to the mail-order pharmacy and ordered the medicine. Two days later, a large box containing a Styrofoam cooler packed with dry ice arrived. The cooler must have measured three feet wide by three feet deep by three feet high, even though the actual package of medication itself, a one month supply of Avonex, was about the size of a small container of ice cream and was less than six inches wide and six inches long. The printed instructions on the medicine package clearly read REFRIG-ERATE IMMEDIATELY.

The following Thursday was the first week of August 2006 and I went by myself to Dr. Blitz's office in East Meadow. I checked in with Dr. Blitz's assistant Donna, and was asked to have a seat. About ten minutes later, Donna escorted me into a private room where Dr. Blitz's Nurse Practitioner, Mary Jean Buhse, greeted me. During the first five minutes I spent with Mary Jean, I quickly became very comfortable with her. She was an energetic, very pleasant young looking middle-aged woman who seemed to know her stuff. She asked about my condition, was cheerful and very personable, quite knowledgeable about MS and offered a lot of compassion and comfort to me. She sensed I was nervous and afraid about recently being diagnosed with MS, so she went out of her way to make me feel at ease. I told Mary Jean the "abridged" version of my story and she seemed genuinely interested and was engaged. She tried her best to ease my fears saying that there were a lot worse things out there, and that doctors and researchers around the world have made significant strides in recent years in the fight against MS to find new treatment options and ultimately a cure. Her comments were indeed comforting. She told me to stay positive, something that I have always remembered and still practice to this day. Almost ten years since having met her, I found Mary Jean to be "spot on" on all fronts.

Mary Jean next described what Avonex was and the importance of minimizing the flu like symptoms by taking Aspirin or Tylenol/Advil prior to injecting. She recommended I take the drug before bedtime. Then came the moment of truth; Mary Jean opened up a package containing a pre-filled syringe (pre-filled with water I correctly assumed, and not with the actual medication), and next opened a desk drawer removing an orange (no, not to eat). She used the orange to demonstrate how the injection should be done, starting with how to hold the needle and explaining how the injection must be made directly into the muscle. Since I was wearing short pants, Mary Jean showed me exactly where the injection could be made, into the top portion of my upper thigh. She placed the orange on my upper thigh, and had me inject the needle into it. I remember the needle being very long. V*ery long*! But since I would be practicing on an orange, "easy-peesy," I thought! Mary Jean then had me practice the procedure on the orange several additional times, until I was comfortable. She also said to be sure I used alternate injection sites each week (i.e. left thigh one week, right thigh the following week, etc.), in order to minimize the occurrence of any injection site reactions and that I could also inject myself on an alternate basis on my left and right buttocks. She also said that I should get into the habit of doing the injection generally the same day and time each week in order to become accustomed to a routine that made it easy to remember to take the medication. She also said it would probably be a good idea to inject myself each week on a Friday or on a Saturday so that in the event I encountered any flu like symptoms, I would have the next day or so off from work to help recover, if needed. Finally, Mary Jean told me to be sure to remove the medication from the refrigerator about thirty minutes prior to injecting so it could warm to room temperature. She went on to say that some people prefer to have a separate person do the injection, and re-emphasized that injecting intramuscularly into the right or left buttocks (along with injecting into the upper portion of either thigh), was fine too.

As I was finishing up my "training" session, Dr. Blitz popped her head into the room for a quick minute to ask how things were going. Both Mary Jean and I let her know that things were going well and that we were just finishing-up. After Dr. Blitz left, Mary Jean told me to feel free and call her if I had any questions or had any difficulties injecting myself with the medication. She also assured me that Dr. Blitz was among the very best MS doctors around, and that I was in good hands. Again, Mary Jean's words were very reassuring and I was quite comfortable after my session with her. Before leaving I thanked her for the support, understanding and words of encouragement.

The next day was Friday, and Luisa and I headed out East for the weekend to our house in the Hamptons. I was sure to take with me a cooler packed with ice and my Avonex MS medication. This weekend would mark the beginning of my journey to treat this horrible disease. Twenty-five years or so earlier, I also was going out to the Hamptons on weekends and bringing with me a cooler packed with ice. Back then though, there was no interferon medication packed inside, just bottles of Budweiser. In 1979, I didn't even know what an interferon was let alone did I know that there was a disease called Multiple Sclerosis. I guess times really do change as you get older!

After dinner I knew it was time. As Mary Jean told me, I took two [extra strength] Tylenol about thirty minutes before doing the deed and I removed the medicine from the refrigerator. Next, I washed my hands thoroughly, waited about a half hour and prepped the injection site by swabbing the upper portion of my right thigh with an alcohol wipe. The plan was for Luisa to "pull the trigger" and give me the injection. As I sat on the edge of a low counter in the master bathroom, I opened the package which contained the pre-filled syringe containing the Avonex. Luisa and I then looked at the needle, gazed at each other and simultaneously said, *"Wow, that needle is f'#^$*%'g huge!"* (An expletive proceeded the word "huge.") As my heart began to race, Luisa held the needle close to my upper thigh and casually said, "Okay, get ready." I closed my eyes and mumbled, "I guess I'm ready." I thought to myself, "Where's the orange?" Luisa then stepped back, turned away, paused and said…, "I can't do this!" Great, I thought as I let out a temporary sigh of relief, thinking momentarily that I was "saved." But then I quickly came back to reality about ten seconds later and knew that if she wasn't going to do it, I would have to. I told her we couldn't put this off any longer and said the time had come. At this point I sensed Luisa's reluctance and hesitation, but she heard me and knew that it was time to proceed. As she moved the syringe closer to my thigh, she took a deep breath. As she was about to "do the deed," I reminded her what Mary Jean said - about how the injection needed to be given intramuscularly. She nodded and placed the cold needle onto my warm thigh which was speckled with goose bumps. We both took deep breaths and as I looked away, Luisa then "pulled the trigger." Surprisingly the injection did not hurt much, and took less than twenty seconds. When finished, Luisa uttered the words "all done." Finally, the anxiety was over. Looking away the entire time with my eyes closed I said, "Done, already? That didn't seem so bad, right?" I wanted to pound my chest now that I was all done with the injection but quickly realized that it was Luisa who did all the work. I was just the pincushion and for me, the anticipation was a lot worse than the injection itself. I knew Luisa felt uneasy about having to do the injection, but I wonder if she really knew how stressful I felt and how anxious I was about being "stuck" with that *BIG f#^$*%'g* needle. If only I could have "bottled" my rapid heartbeat so that she could have gotten the true taste of how nervous and anxious I really was. And I'm sure Luisa's emotions were just as intense (if not more intense) than mine were. Be that as it may, zero hour had come and was now gone. It was the first and to this day the only time that Luisa gave me an injection for my MS. Going forward, I would fly solo!

When the injection was done I proceeded to clean everything up and created a log of the date, time and location on my body of where the needle was given. I remembered what Mary Jean had said about rotating injection sites each week in order to minimize the occurrence of any site reactions. Keeping a log would help me remember to follow her advice. When I was all done cleaning up and creating my log I went into the living room, turned on the Yankee game and collapsed onto the couch. A huge sense of relief set in, as I was all done and didn't have to do this again until the following Friday—a whole week! A few hours later as I went to bed, I took another two Tylenol (as Mary Jean had advised). The next morning when I awoke I felt fine (no flu-like after-effects), and went about my normal routine.

Every Friday thereafter around the same time each evening, I gave myself the Avonex injection. As this was becoming more of a weekly routine, going forward I would always give myself the injections without asking Luisa for her help. I never experienced an issue until about six weeks later when I forgot to take two Tylenol beforehand. Later on that night at around 2 A.M., I awoke from a deep sleep and felt as if I were going to die. I had the chills, felt nauseous and definitely had a fever. My head was pounding, I was sweating profusely and I literally crawled into the bathroom and vomited several times. I remember barely making it to the bathroom before reverse peristalsis sent it. Next I reached into the bathroom cabinet so I could take two Tylenol, crawled back into bed and tried going back to sleep. As I lay in bed wide awake for about two hours afterwards, my mind was racing. My head was pounding, sweat was pouring from my brow and I was burning up. I felt nauseous and the room was spinning. And then finally, I fell back asleep. When I awoke the next morning I felt fine but took another two Tylenol anyway as I was not taking any chances. This would be the first and only time I would forget to "pre and post medicate" when injecting with Avonex. Clearly I learned my lesson, the hard way!

Chapter 7

No Problem, this MS Thing Seems Invisible – Almost!

F or the next year or so, things moved along nicely. I continued with the Avonex injections every Friday, and made sure to take two Tylenol before and after medicating. I guess the horrible flu-like symptoms which I experienced when I initially began taking Avonex taught me a valuable lesson, which I did not care to re-live. Once bitten, twice shy! To be on the safe side, I mentioned my experience to Dr. Blitz and she prescribed a medication called Naproxen just in case I ever forgot to take Tylenol before injecting and needed something quick to help in the middle of the night and ease any flu-like symptoms I might experience.

I saw Dr. Blitz on a quarterly basis throughout 2007, at which time she would order blood tests to be certain the medication prescribed was not having any adverse effects on my blood cells or on my liver. For my first year on the drug, all the bloodwork came back negative and as far as the Avonex went, so far so good. I also had a follow-up MRI done in fall 2007 and the results were basically consistent with the prior scans taken. There were no new lesions so I guess the medication, along with my exercise regimen, was working appropriately. My assessment was that things were going well and that my MS was basically invisible and under control. I had no symptoms and was feeling fine.

Throughout the first half of 2007, I probably did more traveling for work than I could remember since joining Credit Suisse (CS) in 2003. Looking back at my experience in the Residential Mortgage-Backed Securities (RMBS) area, my sudden and increasingly more hectic travel schedule that began in late 2006 probably had something to do with concerns management and outside investors had about CS' portfolio. Hindsight was 20/20; the impending collapse of the mortgage market would soon come about at the end of 2007. Rumblings from investors were beginning to occur in the first quarter of the year concerning the gradual and progressive uptick in losses they were seeing on residential mortgage loans in their bond portfolios. Investors were concerned about how their securitized loans were performing and how their collateral was being managed. One component of my job as a Director supporting the RMBS subprime desk was to go out in the field and visit those entities that were servicing the residential mortgage loans backing the bonds. My visits were focused on identifying any issues and offering recommendations for process change improvements that could help rectify any servicing deficiencies that may have been contributing to some of the losses being experienced by investors. There were approximately one dozen key servicers scattered across the country that required my visiting them, and they serviced approximately 90 percent of the securitized loans backing CS bond issuances.

Looking back now I know the enhanced interest and focus on the Servicing Oversight function was a harbinger of things to come. I mention this because there was an elevated level of investor interest in the servicing function, and a greater sense of urgency for me to visit and call on as many of the key servicers as possible in my role as Director of Servicing Oversight. This elevated level of concern and urgency translated into more scrutiny of my activities from RMBS senior management and traders, who previously showed little interest in my role. Investors too became increasingly more interested. Senior RMBS management frequently asked me to participate in conference calls and attend meetings with outside investors to review their portfolio's asset performance. Hence, more stress! I wasn't used to this as I had acted relatively independently and unmonitored previously in my role with CS. The additional stress associated with this heightened level of interest and scrutiny was new to me, but I really didn't mind. In fact I liked the attention, felt important and genuinely enjoyed the challenge. True, we all know that stress and MS don't get along. Still, even though I had been recently diagnosed with MS, my job performance in no way suffered and I think I handled the added stress without any issues.

The biggest problem I had to deal with when traveling related to carrying the hypodermic needles containing my medication with me each time I went through airport security. The good news was that my business travel only occasionally spanned across weekends and since I gave myself the injections on Friday evenings, I only had to bring my medication with me on an infrequent basis. Storing my medication in checked luggage was not an option, since I usually took with me carry-on baggage only. Besides, even if I did check any luggage the potential for temperature variations below the plane where checked bags were placed was not recommended for transporting any medication, including Avonex. The carry-on of hypodermic needles when boarding airplanes certainly slowed things down. This also presented me with challenges when traveling with others. At that point in time, I had been newly diagnosed and no one was aware (other than Luisa, the girls and maybe one or two other people) that I had MS. So, being pulled aside and questioned by members of the Transportation Security Administration (TSA) to explain why I had needles with me was awkward at times, to say the least. Nonetheless I was able to deal with the TSA and keep my condition hidden from those colleagues that I traveled with.

I'm not sure how I was able to do this, especially at those times when I was traveling with and accompanied by one specific member of my staff in particular (whose name I will not mention). This individual (let's put it this way), was very inquisitive; nosey, one might say, and interested in everybody's business. I always made sure that this individual went ahead of me and passed through airport security first.

Throughout most of 2007 I spent a great deal of time focusing on my work. Spending about nine to ten hours per day at work and traveling quite a bit, I had little free time. I did however, make time to go to the gym a few nights per week when I was in town and was not traveling, and on most Saturdays and Sundays. In addition, on Saturday mornings I began doing physical therapy (or PT) for vestibular training (even though I was not experiencing any noticeable balance issues at the time). Dr. Gottesaman had mentioned this to me as an option to consider, although he did not actually specifically recommend it. Still though I figured it couldn't hurt, so I asked the doctor for a script. At that time, PT visits under my medical insurance plan (once approved) were unlimited, with a six-dollar co-pay; five years later PT visits under my medical insurance plan became capped, required pre-approval after six visits and had a fifty dollar co-pay. I figured that being as active as possible was probably a good thing. Was I clairvoyant or what?

Whenever I did travel for business, I would bring along with me a set of workout clothes and try to get in an exercise session or two at the fitness center in the hotel that I was staying at. I enjoyed working out plus I knew it was something recommended for patients having MS. Little did I know how critical exercise would become in helping me deal with the disease in the years ahead.

In early September 2007 I was getting a strong feeling that the residential mortgage loan securitization business was in trouble, as losses at CS were beginning to mount. I sensed that senior management would be looking at headcount and would likely consider doing some reductions to the workforce, especially since mortgage loan origination volume was declining and the RMBS unit in which I worked was more than sufficiently staffed. Some might have said the RMBS unit was over-staffed; in hindsight, it probably was. CS' RMBS business employed about three hundred fulltime professionals, was part of the much larger Fixed Income business and produced record profits of nearly $1 billion in the prior year (2006). While I knew that some workforce reductions were likely, I never expected what was about to happen and that the reductions would directly impact me. After all, a large part of my responsibilities related to the oversight of third parties responsible for servicing loans for CS investors and bond holders. If anything, CS investors placed a high level of importance on the Servicing Oversight function, and were accordingly very supportive of it. The recent increased level of attention and focus on the Servicing Oversight role gave me assurance that I was insulated from any upcoming workforce reductions. This, coupled with the fact that senior CS management touted Servicing Oversight as a selling point to attract investors to participate in new deals, was surely a "clincher." It was no secret that the Servicing Oversight role gave investors a high level of confidence that their concerns and interests in RMBS were being addressed. As such, this was often a decisive determining factor in an investor's decision to participate in a securitization issue and become a new or remain an existing "customer" of the firm. And maintaining and increasing the overall number of new and existing customers doing business with CS was critical to RMBS' overall success and profitability, especially in a period of declining loan origination volume. So it seemed only logical that the Servicing Oversight function which I managed was critical, and as such was entirely safe from workforce reductions—right? *WRONG!*

While I suspected I may be asked to contribute and offer one or two names to the headcount reduction roster, what came next was devastating. Late one Thursday afternoon in the fall of 2007, I was called into the COO's office and told some shocking news: "Your job, along with the jobs of everyone on your entire team, is being eliminated. Today will be everyone's last day, including you. Assigned Human Resource professionals will meet individually with everyone, including you, to review and discuss severance packages that will be given in accordance with position level and length of service. They will then walk everyone back to their desks to oversee them as they pack their personal belongings and then escort them out of the building." I was stunned! I asked the reason why the Servicing Oversight group was being eliminated, but was not provided with any real and substantive rationale. I was not shy in sharing my opinion with the COO that I felt the decision was shortsighted and the wrong thing to do. The COO listened and I got the sense he agreed with my opinion, although he did not directly come out and say so. It didn't matter though as the decision had already been made and would stand. After pausing for a moment or two, I slowly rose from my seat, shook his hand, said goodbye and left his office. I returned to my desk and called Luisa to let her know what had just happened. Shocked, she asked why. I told her that I didn't want to get into the details over the phone and that I would explain things to her later when I got home. I asked if she would mind picking me up and driving into the city to come get me, which she agreed to do. Luisa arrived at my office on 23rd and Madison in NYC about ninety minutes later. A few days later I learned that about sixty percent of CS' RMBS work force, or about one hundred eighty people, were included in this round of workforce reductions. It was not just me and my group of nearly twenty professionals that were given the boot. By the end of the year, CS would lay-off another forty people in the RMBS unit, bringing the total number of workforce reductions made in 2006 to over two hundred, or about seventy percent of the group.

Despite losing my job I was confident that I would quickly find employment, given my background, skills, education, experience and vast professional network. My six months of severance pay gave me some added comfort and cushion and I believed that things would be okay. This was only the second time in my career that I became the victim of a workforce reduction (the other time being in 2002 when I was with Citibank, and was laid off as a result of the merger with Traveler's Insurance and Solomon Smith Barney). While devastated after being employed with Citibank for nearly sixteen years and uncertain as to what lie ahead, I was able to land a senior level job at Credit Suisse within six months of being laid off. In fact, my new position at CS would prove to be financially more lucrative than was my prior role at Citi. So with that as a backdrop, I was less concerned I would be out of a job for any significant length of time this go-around. However, little did I know the magnitude of the financial collapse about to hit the financial market at the end of 2007, the impact this would have on the U.S. employment market and the difficulty I would encounter finding work. The stress associated with not working and looking for a job would only increase in the weeks and months that followed. Luckily though I was able to cope well, and again my MS was virtually unaffected. I was beginning to think that having MS was pretty benign since I had no real symptoms. I was feeling pretty confident with Dr. Blitz's decision to have me start treatment so quickly, and was sure this was helping to keep my affliction under control. That, along with my newfound friend "Gym" and the weekly PT routines I had started, must have been positively impacting my overall well-being.

As part of my severance, I was given a pretty benevolent outplacement package. Being a Director of the firm, I was provided with six months of outplacement service. My guess was that as a CS Director, the outplacement service benefit may have been given for a longer time-frame but was capped due to my relatively short five year tenure with them. The day after my separation from CS, I called the outplacement office and spoke with the advisor assigned to me. I made arrangements to meet with him the following Monday, despite his recommendation that I take a week or so off to "relax" and collect my thoughts. I respectfully declined and told him that I wanted to see him the following Monday to start outplacement so I could immediately begin looking for a new job. I was eager to commence my job search and approached outplacement as if it were a fulltime profession. In my mind I didn't want to think about relaxing until I landed a job. When that occurred, I would have a clearer head and could plan on taking a week off prior to starting any new position.

For the next several months, I would come into the outplacement center located in New York City near Grand Central Station four days per week. I would arrive at the outplacement center each morning (Monday through Thursday) when it opened at 8 A.M., and would generally leave around 5:30 P.M. On most days I was the first person to get there and had to wait for the office manager to arrive and unlock the front door. In the evening I was usually one of the last people to leave, and often greeted the cleaning people on my way out. I took off on Fridays to "play" unless I was fortunate enough to land an interview in the city on those days. The outplacement center helped me to further expand my network and provided me with an office, use of a dedicated computer, a telephone and an assigned counselor that would meet with me every Monday morning. The counselor was also available throughout the week to answer any questions that I may have had and to provide advice. The center also offered at least one or two information "training" seminars each week which I generally attended, about how best to conduct a meaningful job search. For nearly five months, I networked intensely and probably had more coffee and lunch meetings than I could count. And yes, I was able to land several interviews. Looking for a *job* had become a *fulltime job*! Unfortunately, the latter part of 2007 through 2009 was probably the worst time to be in the market looking for work. I quickly began to realize this.

After speaking with an old friend (Allen Gutterman) on and off for about five months, we decided to give some serious thought to starting a business. The then current job environment really gave me pause to stop and think about doing something on my own. Like me, Allen was a twenty plus year veteran of the mortgage finance industry. And like me, he saw the mortgage market imploding almost daily. Together with a few other professionals, Allen and I saw that there was a need to provide advisory services to banks and other third parties (like insurance companies, pension funds, etc.) to help recover losses they had sustained due to various misrepresentations made by originators and sellers of mortgage paper. These misrepresentations (right out "lies" in many cases) influenced and convinced them to invest and purchase mortgage-backed bonds. In the spring of 2008, Allen, myself and three others formed an advisory and consulting firm called Recourse Recovery Management Services, or RRMS Advisors. We quickly began soliciting new clients to get business. Allen, who was President and CEO of a separate recruiting firm, had office space on 39th Street off Madison Avenue and had some empty cubicles which we could use.

As I was about nearing the end of the outplacement services provided to me as part of my severance package from CS, I would slightly change my commuting routine. Instead of going into the outplacement center in NYC, I would go to the 39th Street office. Still, I only commuted into the city four days per week and continued to hold Friday's as my "play day" (barring any new or pressing business issues, or even interviews). Although I was actively soliciting new business opportunities for RRMS, I continued to network in the hopes of landing a fulltime job just in case the new business didn't work out. While I was serious about building the business with Allen, I still kept my options open and continued to explore the market for potential job opportunities. Since being laid-off from CS six months earlier, I probably interviewed with about a dozen or so companies. Unfortunately, none of my interviews ever materialized into a fulltime job, as the U.S. mortgage and financial markets continued to worsen almost by the day. Plus, no one was interested in hiring an almost fifty something middle aged man having over twenty-five years of experience and with salary requirements commensurate with the tenure of a former Wall Street executive. It worked out well for me though in the end, as not being able to land a regular fulltime job only helped me focus more on building and growing RRMS. It also helped me to better manage and cope with my MS.

I remember one of the last interviews I had in June 2008 and rushing from 39th Street and Madison Avenue to 51st Street and 6th Avenue for a 1 P.M. appointment. In my haste to get to the interview on-time, I tripped and fell to the ground. I sustained a bruised and slightly bloodied face. Rushing and about two blocks from my destination, I remember after tripping and falling to the ground being helped up by a passersby. When I came to my feet I brushed myself off, thanked the person who helped me get up and walked briskly to the building where my interview was scheduled. I remember navigating around a construction zone where work was being done outside the building I was going to, checking-in at the front desk in the lobby, taking the elevator upstairs and paying a visit first to the men's room to try and clean up my face. Luckily the bleeding was not that bad and had virtually stopped before my interview was scheduled to begin. However, the bruises and scrapes on my face were noticeable. I was also fortunate that I did not rip my suit. I went into my interview, which was with two senior partners in New York, and one senior partner in Washington, D.C., who participated via video conference. I remember an Administrative Assistant escorting me into a conference room; luckily for me, she was having trouble setting up the connection for the video conference. So the start of the interview was delayed for nearly twenty minutes. She apologized for the delay, and I excused myself and went back to the restroom to dab my "wounds" in an attempt to look as presentable as possible for the interview. I walked back into the conference room and shortly thereafter the two partners that I would be interviewing with in-person had arrived. The video hook-up with the D.C. office was finally established, and the interview began. In my opening remarks I recall apologizing for my appearance and said that I had tripped on a construction grate in front of the building (I stretched the truth a bit), fell and bruised my face. I figured I would come right out in the open and start-off with my story in case the partners interviewing me wondered why my face was bruised. After my opening remarks, the partners apologized and asked if I had hurt myself. The two partners in the New York office immediately began to complain and voice their concerns about the hazardous construction conditions around the front entrance to the building. They continued apologizing profusely that I had tripped and fallen, were quite upset that my interview with them was to blame for my fall and wanted to be certain that I was not hurt. They could not have been more apologetic; I guess they were worried that I might turn around and file a law suit against the company! Boy, did I feel guilty. ("Wow," I thought to myself, "I turned a near disaster into an empathetic interview where the firm's senior partners took personal responsibility for my mishap. If for nothing else, this should have made them feel guilty enough to offer me the job.") By the way, while the interview went very well, it never did result in a formal job offer. The experience though was quite memorable.

I never really thought about how and why I tripped and fell, and never even remotely thought it had anything to do with my having MS. Back then I was sure it did not. But looking back now, I wonder if it really did. I question if the clumsiness and tripping Luisa noted a few years earlier that eventually drove me to see a doctor ultimately leading to my diagnosis of MS was really to blame. I guess I'll never know. In any event, up until this point MS continued to be fairly benign and invisible. I was not experiencing any real symptoms other than feeling tired toward the end of most days and not being able to tolerate any extreme heat or humidity. Since I was approaching fifty, I just shrugged off the fatigue and attributed my heat intolerance to "old age."

By the middle of 2008 I essentially halted my efforts to explore job opportunities and go on interviews. I became focused more exclusively on building the RRMS business. In teaming-up with three other professionals, Allen and I had some initial success attracting clients and soliciting new business. Cash flow was challenging though, as dividing the profits (which were not much in the beginning) amongst five people did not leave much cash for each partner. Two years later in early 2010, we actually parted ways with two of the other partners. Presently, only myself, Allen and Brian are the three remaining founding partners of RRMS Advisors.

Around September 2008 I began to notice I was walking with a slight limp. While I thought it was very slight, it must have been noticeable because on occasion people would ask why I was limping. My response would be to say I had hurt my knee or that I was breaking-in a new pair of shoes. I would then quickly change the subject and move on. Now, whenever I visited my mom she would surely ask why I was limping. By this point in time she had been diagnosed with osteoporosis and ulcerative colitis. These ailments, along with her existing heart condition of atrial fibrillation, prompted me to visit her with greater frequency. Now that I was actually limping, I could no longer deny it and tell her that I was not. So I would convey to my mom that I had hurt my knee whenever she asked. And she always did ask! My mom would always tell me to go see a doctor to get checked out. She would not only tell me that each time I saw her, but she would call me at least once a week and ask if I had made an appointment to see a doctor for my knee. I felt terrible lying to her, but figured she had enough to worry about with her own ailments and caring for my father without me adding to the mix. So, I continued with my fabricated "story."

Throughout 2008 I continued to see Dr. Blitz quarterly and get my blood checked. In October 2008, she ordered a follow-up MRI. I received a copy of the written laboratory report which revealed that "there was no enhancement of the existing demyelinating plaques, but that there was however plaque noted on the right parietal lobe which did not show on the test results from the prior year's examination." That may have explained why I started to limp. But, who knows. Nonetheless I needed to discuss this further with Dr. Blitz. In my next appointment with her I would be sure to ask about this. In November 2008 I went for bloodwork ordered by Dr. Blitz. Usually I would have to call for the test results. But in late November 2008, Mary Jean from Dr. Blitz's office called me and said that I needed to stop taking Avonex immediately since my bilirubin level was extremely elevated. (I thought to myself, "Billy Reuben, wasn't that the name of a kid that I played stickball with when I was growing up in Queens?") I asked Mary Jean what an elevated bilirubin level meant and she told me that it signified that my liver enzymes were high, likely as a result of taking Avonex and that I needed to stop taking the medication immediately. "You need to stop taking Avonex and be off it for at least one month before you can begin a new treatment," Mary Jean told me. She asked that I make an appointment to see Dr. Blitz to review my recent MRI and bloodwork results and to discuss alternative treatment options. This would also be the time for me to tell the doctor about my limp. Unfortunately, the holidays were rapidly approaching and I was unable to schedule an appointment with Dr. Blitz until after the New Year.

It wasn't until the first week of January 2009 that I was able to schedule an appointment with Dr. Blitz. I had been off Avonex for slightly over one month and was ready to discuss my condition with her as well as starting a new alternative treatment. When I was finally able to get an appointment with Dr. Blitz, I told her about my limp that started to occur in the late summer/early fall of 2008. After she asked me a series of questions about how I was feeling, Dr. Blitz exerted downward pressure separately on both my arms and legs as I pushed up. She then asked me to kick (or extend) and retract each leg separately while I was in a seated position. When I was done, she told me she noted some tightness, stiffness and some slight weakness with the muscle (and muscle tone) in my left leg. She told me that this was likely impacting my gait, causing me to limp and my foot to drop. She then asked me to walk down the hall, watching and timing me as I did. When I returned back to her desk Dr. Blitz wrote me a prescription for Baclofen, a drug designed to help with spasticity, or muscle tightness/stiffness. She told me that I should take two pills per day—one in the morning and the other at bedtime. I then told Dr. Blitz that other than my limp, the only other thing I noticed of late was that I was feeling much more tired toward the end of each day. Dr. Blitz listened and then explained a bit more about the results of my most recent MRI. She referenced the formal written lab report and said that there was one small additional area of plaque noted on the right lobe of my brain, but that there were no other appreciable changes appearing on this MRI in comparison to the prior scan. Nonetheless though, a new lesion appeared. I was not happy.

Dr. Blitz then said that since I had been off Avonex for nearly five weeks, it was time to take another blood test to check my liver enzyme level. "Assuming your liver enzymes have normalized, I would like you to begin taking Betaseron, which requires injection every other day." Dr. Blitz went on to tell me that like Avonex, Betaseron was in the interferon class of drugs, that flu-like side-effects were common when starting the drug but that these symptoms generally stopped about a week or two after starting treatment. As a precaution and to protect against any flu-like symptoms, she told me I should take Aspirin or Tylenol (as I did when I took Avonex), but only for the first few weeks when I began taking the drug. She went on to indicate that once approved, a representative from the drug company would be calling me to schedule an in-home visit to show me how to prepare and administer the drug. Unlike Avonex, Betaseron needed to be mixed. Additionally unlike Avonex, this medication was administered with an injector pen. Plus, the needles were much smaller. She also indicated that blood tests needed to be done quarterly to check my liver enzymes to be sure the drug was not causing any adverse impacts.

With respect to my limp and foot drop, Dr. Blitz gave me a script for a drug called 4-AP Fampradine which at that time needed to be filled at a compound pharmacy and taken twice a day and twelve hours apart; once in the morning and once in the evening to avoid the possibility of seizures. (4-AP would later come to market as Ampyra, and become better known as the "MS Walking Drug.") In terms of my tiredness, Dr. Blitz gave me a script for a drug called Provigil that was on the market and designed to treat narcolepsy. It had been shown to boost overall energy levels for people having MS. The Provigil prescription called for me to take one pill each morning after breakfast. I filled both prescriptions later that day, and began taking 4-AP Fampradine that evening and Provigil the next morning. Dr. Blitz also suggested I consider starting a steroid infusion of a drug called Solu-Medrol. The infusion, which would be done in her office and be given monthly, would be stopped after six consecutive monthly treatments. Each infusion would take about an hour. Then in another six months the infusions could commence again for an additional six consecutive rounds until complete. When I asked why the "on-again/off-again" infusion treatment regimen, Dr. Blitz indicated that Solu-Medrol was an anti-inflammatory corticosteroid. If taken for prolonged periods of time, corticosteroids were known to cause bone weakness that could potentially lead to osteoporosis. Dr. Blitz recommended I try it, and went on to tell me that the only other side-effect of Solu-Medrol may be an increase in appetite and a bitter or unpleasant taste in my mouth at the time of infusion. She told me that the benefit of taking it would be a reduction in inflammation caused by the MS and provide me with a resultant surge in my overall energy level. This sounded good to me, so I told her I'd try it and would call her administrative assistant Donna to schedule my first infusion appointment.

In the interim, I began taking both the Baclofen and Provigil pills she had prescribed. After a few days of taking both drugs, I did not notice any change in my gait but did however notice that my left leg was not as tight as it was previously. But, I continued to limp and experience foot drop. I did however, keep taking the Baclofen. Regarding the fatigue I felt toward the end of each day, I noticed I had more energy and felt less tired since I began taking Provigil. I called and told this to Dr. Blitz, at which time she apprised me that the results of the bloodwork taken earlier during the week showed that my liver enzymes were back to within a normal range. She then gave me the green light to start taking Betaseron. As I was told by Dr. Blitz, a representative from the drug company did contact me and came to my home to "train" me on how to mix and administer the drug. Unlike Avonex which was injected intramuscularly one time per week, Beteseron injections needed to be administered every other day and done subcutaneously. As Betaseron did not come in a pre-mixed vial, the fact that I had to "prepare" it at first seemed like it would be a nuisance. However after a few injections, I got the hang of it and preparing the drug and administering it did not present any real issues. I alternated injection sites as recommended during "training," and used the injector pen provided to administer the drug. The good thing was that since the injections were done subcutaneously and with an injector pen, administering the drug was quite simple and virtually painless. And now that I had stopped taking Avonex, I no longer needed to inject myself weekly with a huge hypodermic needle deep into the outer thigh muscle of my leg or into my buttocks!

A few weeks went by and I had no ill-effects or flu-like symptoms from taking Betaseron. By this point I had stopped taking Tylenol before and after each injection. "Easy-peesy," I thought to myself. After all, I was now an expert at giving myself MS injections. This was a far cry from the angst and stress which I felt the very first time I injected myself with Avonex. I was still limping slightly, but I did notice a boost in my overall energy level. I was going into my office in the New York City four days per week and overall, things seemed to be going okay. I continued frequenting the gym about four times per week and was going to PT every Saturday morning. Having my own business gave me more scheduling flexibility and more free time than I would have had otherwise if I were working for a large corporation. Things like scheduling doctor's appointments, taking lab tests and working-out at the gym were much easier for me and much less of a hassle.

The next week in early March 2009 I scheduled my first infusion of Solu-Medrol at Dr. Blitz's office. This followed a surprise fiftieth birthday party that Luisa and my daughters had thrown for me at my house the prior Saturday night. The party was great, as it gave me a chance to connect with old friends and reminisce about the "good old days." My parents were there too, and yes, you guessed it - my mom asked about my limp. I shrugged it off as usual and proceeded to change the subject. The following Monday was steroid time! The Solu-Medrol infusion took about an hour, and Mary Jean was great as she walked me through the entire procedure. She gave me some hard candies to suck on throughout the infusion to counteract the bitter taste in my mouth that I was experiencing. That evening, I went to the gym as usual. This time though I literally felt like superman, as I was able to bench-press more weight and do more exercise repetitions than I was able to do previously. In many respects I was feeling almost "super-human." Now I knew why athletes took steroids and other performance enhancing drugs. The funny thing was that I was no longer limping (or thought I

95

wasn't). "This is great," I thought to myself, and wondered how long this super human feeling would last. I only wished that I felt like this the prior Saturday night after my surprise birthday party when everyone left my house and I was helping Luisa clean up.

About five days later, the effects of the steroids wore off and I was back to feeling my "normal" self. That wasn't so bad, as I really had no complaints and always reminded myself that things could certainly be a whole lot worse. I began noticing my limp again, but felt that overall my MS was somewhat invisible and not a big deal. My biggest area of focus now was on procuring new business for RRMS and maximizing my personal cash flow. Also my mom was in and out of the hospital throughout the first part of 2009, first undergoing treatment for her ulcerative colitis and separately for a rapid and irregular heartbeat caused by atrial fibrillation. On top of this, osteoporosis was playing havoc on her lower back and the pain she had as a result of having a fractured vertebrae made it increasingly more difficult for her to walk. Each time I would stop by the house to see mom or to pay her a visit to see her in the hospital she would always ask me if I had seen a doctor regarding my limp. Like always I shrugged it off, but at one point I remember telling my mom that she really needed to concentrate on herself getting better and not worry so much about me. Still though, she would not give up. She even went as far to pull my father aside at one point and asked him to speak with me in private. I recall my father saying, "Your mother wants to know why you are limping and if you have seen a doctor." I chuckled and thought to myself just how persistent she was in trying to find out about my health. I then told my father to let my mom know that I would be scheduling an appointment to see a doctor soon.

Then the following month, something strange happened. It was on a Saturday morning during the second week of April 2009 when my neighbor Steve, who had two extra tickets to a baseball game that afternoon at the new Yankee Stadium, asked if my daughter Lauren (who is a HUGE Yankee fan) and I wanted to go with him. I immediately jumped on the offer as both Lauren and I were dying to see the new stadium. I remember it being an unusually hot day for that time of the year. The high temperature hit the low nineties that early mid-April afternoon. Steve drove to the game and we parked the car in the indoor lot across the street from the old stadium. It was about a two block walk to the new stadium and the three of us made our way over. As we did, I noticed that my left leg was tight and would not allow me to bend my knee as I walked. As a result, I limped and struggled to make it to the new stadium and by the time we got there I could barely walk. The heat did not help either. Finally after about a half hour, we were inside the stadium and made it to our seats. While not in the upper deck, the seats were not on ground level either. They were however, up one tier. Thank goodness our seats were a few rows from the front of the section; had they been up any further, I do not think I could have made it. Lauren and my neighbor Steve continued to ask if I was okay and what was wrong. I told them I had sprained my knee and that I would be okay. Before the game started we were all very eager to visit Monument Park, which was at the complete opposite end of the stadium near the outfield. Luckily (for me), Monument Park was closed due to the huge crowd of people on line to visit it. As a result the following message from Bob Sheppard came over the stadium's public address system:

> *"Ladies and gentlemen, may I have your attention please. Due to the large number of fans currently in queue for Monument Park, the Yankees have regretfully halted visitation beyond those patrons currently in line. We apologize for any inconvenience, and hope that you patronize Monument Park during a future visit to Yankee Stadium. Thank you."*

Boy, I thought to myself, was I lucky. What timing! There was no possibility of me navigating my way to the outfield area on the other side of the stadium where Monument Park was located. And, it would be the last time that I would hear Bob Sheppard's iconic voice in person! He retired the following year and passed away in 2010.

When the game ended (I don't even recall if the Yankees won or lost), we began making our way to the exit toward the parking lot. By this point I was very hot, very tired, very wobbly, had trouble keeping my balance. I could barely walk. I'm sure sitting in the hot sun for several hours didn't help. My left leg was totally stiff (or spastic), and I could barely bend my left knee. As we slowly made our way out of the ballpark, my mind was racing and I was thinking the worst. Thoughts that crossed my mind included: "Would I be able to walk again?" "Will this mean I'll be confined to a wheelchair for the rest of my life?" "How will I be able to work?" "How would I go up and down the stairs in my house?" "How would I tell Deanna and Lauren that I couldn't walk?" These and many other thoughts raced throughout my mind during all nine innings of the game as I sat in the hot sun. Needless to say what was supposed to be a great and memorable experience in my first visit to the new Yankee Stadium was a far from that. What a terrible day! In leaving the stadium, what should have been at most a ten-minute walk from the stands to my neighbor Steve's car in the parking garage took nearly thirty minutes. As I walked down the stadium ramps toward the exit, I was very unsteady and felt as if I were drunk. All along the walk until we reached the car, I held onto every wall, railing, lamp post, etc. to prevent me from tripping and falling. When we finally reached the car and I opened the door, I plopped right down on the passenger's seat and immediately asked Steve to turn on the AC full blast! "Wow," I thought to myself, "this sucks. I never before felt this way."

After a fifty-minute drive home we arrived back to our house in Jericho and I was feeling better. My drunken, wobbly feeling was gone.

I'm sure the cool air that was blasting from the AC really helped me "revive." Sitting for nearly three hours under the hot sun in the stands at Yankee Stadium certainly contributed to my situation. At one point in the afternoon I think the temperature reached ninety-two degrees (at least that's what scoreboard in center field displayed). This temperature was pretty unheard of for a day in the middle of April. I always heard that MS and heat didn't mix well, but now I knew for sure they do not. When I got into the driveway of my house and my neighbor Steve dropped Lauren and me off, I stood up and noticed I had less stiffness in my left leg and no longer felt as if I were drunk. I was able to walk into the house without holding on to anything. Still slightly limping, I felt a lot better and quite rejuvenated from how I had felt earlier that afternoon. Nonetheless I would be certain to call Dr. Blitz after the weekend was over on Monday to tell her what had happened. Luisa reinforced that plan of action too.

I spoke with Dr. Blitz the following Monday, explained what happened, and she told me that I probably had an exacerbation. She said she wanted me to go on seven straight days of Solu-Medrol steroid infusions. Dr. Blitz then went on to tell me that a nurse would be contacting me in the afternoon and make arrangements to come to my house with the medication and an intravenous pole. "At home infusions—why?" I asked. "Yes," Dr. Blitz replied. "It makes more sense that way, instead of having you come into the office for seven straight days. Besides, on days when our office is closed, like Saturday and Sunday, you will still need to have the infusions." She went on to tell me that when I was done with the Solu-Medrol infusions she wanted me to take the oral steroid Prednisone consecutively for the following seven days, and have me titrate the dosage throughout that period. She said that the nurse coming to my house would also be bringing me the Prednisone script and advising me how to administer it.

After the nurse had come to the house, placed a port in my right forearm for me to administer the infusions and showed me exactly how to give myself the drug daily over the next seven days, I was all set. For the next seven consecutive days I gave myself the Solu-Medrol infusions each night after dinner time. To do so, I would remove a drip bag from my refrigerator, let it sit on the counter for about forty minutes before using it to allow it to warm to room temperature, hook it up to the intravenous pole the nurse left with me and start the infusion. After administering the infusions for seven straight days, I began taking the Prednisone pills and titrating the dosage (i.e. I would take seven pills on day seven, six pills on day six, five pills on day five, etc.). Throughout the two weeks that I was on steroids, I was eating everything in sight. My weight soared nearly twelve pounds to one hundred eighty. I was feeling very hyperactive and I had tons of energy. I felt great! Most nights I found myself lying in bed and wide awake by 3:00 A.M., tossing, turning and trying to fall back asleep. Most days I could not get back to sleep so I'd head off to the gym when it opened at 7 A.M. Once I got there I would do my normal workout in less than an hour. Prior to taking the steroids, my workout generally took about an hour and ten minutes. Now I was even adding between ten and twenty pounds of weight onto every piece of universal gym equipment that I used. To boot there were even a couple of days when I'd go back to the gym later in that same evening. For the two weeks that I was on steroids and for about three weeks afterwards, I was no longer limping, did not have foot drop and had no spasticity at all in my left leg. And my fatigue was now a thing of the past. I had more energy than I knew what to do with! "This was great," I thought to myself.

The week after I stopped taking the Prednisone I had an appointment to see Dr. Blitz. On my way to her office I finally dropped off the intravenous pole at the nurse's office (albeit two weeks late and prompted by two separate reminder telephone messages left on my home answering machine). My visit with Dr. Blitz was quick. I was in and out of her office in less than fifteen minutes, as she just wanted to see how I was doing and watch me walk. As I was about to leave, Dr. Blitz ran an idea by me about going off Betaseron and considering changing therapies. She mentioned to me a drug that had been in use for a couple of years called Tysabri, and said it was given via a ninety-minute intravenous infusion once a month. Because the infusion was not continuous and needed to be halted on occasion while being administered in order to check one's blood pressure and pulse, the elapsed time spent at the infusion center during each sitting would be several hours. Still though, the once-per-month thing really piqued my interest as I would no longer need to be bothered by mixing a drug and injecting myself every other day. My interest level quickly fell though as Dr. Blitz told me about one potentially rare side-effect of the drug. She went on to say that a very small number cases had occurred where patients taking Tysabri developed something called Progressive Multifocal Leukoencephalopathy, or PML. "What is PML?" I asked. Dr. Blitz told me that PML is a rare and potentially fatal brain infection; it usually leads to death or severe disability. "Oh, is that all?" I sarcastically thought to myself. "Where do I sign up?"

Without hesitation I told her, "No thanks, I'm not interested. I think I'll stay on Beteseron." Dr. Blitz gave me some literature on Tysabri and told me to read through it at my leisure and give it some thought. She said that MS patients on Tysabri had fewer flare-ups (or exacerbations) and that there was evidence in clinical trials that use of the drug resulted in slower disability progression in comparison to the other MS therapies on the market. I took the literature and told Dr. Blitz I would read through it but that I didn't think changing to Tysabri was for me, especially given the potential for developing a fatal brain infection. I left her office and worked from home the remainder of that day. I may have glanced briefly through the materials she gave me, but given the possibility of developing PML I had no intention of switching to Tysabri. Eventually I threw away the literature she had given to me. Driving home, I felt great and actually had thoughts of returning to Yankee Stadium at a later date. This time though, I would be sure to sit out of the sun or attend a night game, but I didn't. In actuality, nearly seven years would go by until I would actually return to Yankee Stadium.

That following summer was a non-event for me as far as MS went. After a few weeks of taking the steroids, I had pretty much returned to my old self. Yes, after a while, I began to limp a bit more and the spasticity in my left leg had begun to rear its ugly head again, but ever so slightly (although it was slowly worsening). Foot drop was back too, and I had to have most of my pants tailored so that the waste lines could be let out to accommodate all of the weight that I had gained from taking the steroids. Overall though, I was fine. About two months later I called Dr. Blitz to tell her about the increase in tightness I had in my left leg. She raised my Baclofen dosage from two pills per day to four, calling in a new script to my pharmacy. After a few days of taking the new dosage, the muscles in my left leg, while still somewhat tight, felt a bit looser than before I increased the Baclofen dosage. I was now taking four Baclofen pills per day.

Throughout the next few months, my condition remained relatively unchanged. Once each quarter I had bloodwork done and no issues were noted. In August 2009 I went in for a follow-up MRI that showed no new lesions had formed, and that those lesions that previously existed were consistent and unchanged from the prior scan. I continued receiving Solu-Medrol infusions in accordance with the six month "on-again/off-again" regimen that Dr. Blitz had prescribed. Each month for about five days after getting the steroid infusions, I had a very high energy level and felt like Hercules. This inspired me to workout at the gym more frequently. It was also during those weeks that I would do more things around the house, like cleaning out the garage and reorganizing pantry cabinets, etc. These were all things that I had put off doing in prior months. Luisa was happy about that! About a week after each steroid treatment, my energy level would return to "normal." The muscles in my left leg would begin to tighten and on occasion my leg would spasm causing me to wake up in the middle of the night. As the months went by, the overall level of stiffness and spasticity in my left leg slowly increased. At one of my check-ups with Dr. Blitz she increased my Baclofen dosage again, this time from four to six pills per day. While this helped reduce some of the spasticity, it also caused me to feel more tired toward the end of each day. I learned that one of the side-effects of taking Baclofen was an increase in fatigue.

My mom had been in and out of hospitals for the better part of September and October 2009 for treatment of diverticulitis and osteoporosis. At one point in early October, her ability to walk had been significantly compromised and the doctors recommended she be moved from a hospital to a rehabilitation center. Now that her diverticulitis was somewhat under control and the lower back pain she was experiencing as a result of her osteoporosis had slightly lessened, rehab was recommended so she could "learn to walk" again. I would visit my mom nearly every day while she was in the rehab center, and almost every time I saw her she would ask again about my limp and if I had seen a doctor. And every time she would ask, I would tell her not to worry about me and to focus on doing what the clinicians and doctors told her so that she could get better, be discharged and get home in time for Thanksgiving. I remember visiting her one day in early November 2009. During my visit with her, my mom was going on about the New York Yankees who had just won the World Series. I remember my mom, who had become a big Yankee fan over the years, saying to me, "Boy, that Derek Jeter is something else. Did you hear that they now call him Mr. November?"

A few days later on November 12, 2009, I got a phone call at work in the morning that my mom's heart was beating rapidly and that she was having difficulty breathing. Funny because when I saw her the day before, she seemed fine. I was told that the doctors who were attending to her at the rehab center were currently assessing her condition and would shortly be determining whether or not she should be transferred to a hospital. I was torn between whether or not I should leave the office and go see her or wait until the doctor at the rehab center called me back. I decided to remain in my Manhattan office and wait for the doctor's call. I quickly phoned Luisa to tell her what was happening. After hanging up the telephone with me, she immediately rushed over to the rehab center to see her. Less than two hours later, the head doctor from the rehab center called me offering condolences and said that say my mom had passed away from respiratory distress. I was devastated!

Shocked and distraught, I dropped back into my chair and sobbed uncontrollably. Just like that, my mom was gone. What a shock. Never again would she ask about my limp and bug me to see a doctor. And never again would she talk to me about "Mr. November." I cried for the good part of an hour. One consolation was that Luisa was there when she died. I had nearly forgotten that my mom was also suffering from atrial fibrillation, so her passing from cardiac arrest was somewhat of a surprise. My mom was eighty-four years young when she died.

At the time I got the call, my partners Allen and Brian were there to console me, with Allen going so far as to get his car from a nearby parking garage from where he lived in Manhattan and drive me to my dad's house in Queens so that I could tell him the devastating news in person. After I was able to somewhat contain my emotions, Brian helped me down the elevator from the office to the street and helped me get into Allen's car. By this point in time Allen had retrieved his car from a nearby parking garage and double-parked in front of the building. On the car ride into Queens, I phoned my brother. Trying to compose my emotions, I told him what had happened and indicated to him that I was on my way to dad's house. I remember him taking a long pause and in a choked up voice him saying, "I'm on my way to the house, and will meet you there."

When I got to my dad's house my brother and his wife Debbie were outside waiting for me to arrive. I remember us all crying. As we were about to go inside to my dad's house, Luisa pulled up arriving from the rehab center where she was with my mom when she passed away. The four of us, after composing ourselves went inside together to tell my dad the sad news...that his partner of over sixty-two years, our mom, had passed away. I think either Luisa or myself broke the news to him that mom had died. When dad heard the news he immediately fell back into his easy chair and began to cry. We all cried. Luisa tried to console him by saying that she was there with mom at the end. It made no difference though. Dad continued to cry uncontrollably, and began blaming himself for agreeing to send her to the rehabilitation center and not have her come home to receive the therapy she needed. We were all crying—it was very sad. Dad would never again be himself. How very heartbreaking!

For nearly five years until dad passed away in 2014, not a day would go by when we spoke that he would say, "I should have never agreed to send her to that *f'#%$&*'g* [expletive] rehab place. I should have insisted she come home and have someone come to the house each day and give her therapy. Your mother would still be alive today if I didn't send her there." Each time he would say this, either I or someone in the family would tell him it wasn't his fault and that he needed to stop blaming himself. It was no use. My dad was convinced that my mother's passing was his fault, and his actions were to blame for her death.

After the wake and the funeral service was over, I was still in shock. Dealing with such a dramatic situation and now having to worry endlessly about my dad did cause a "*little* bit" of stress. Just a *little*, to say the least. I had heard that like the hot and humid weather, stress was not a friend to MS either. It took me a few months to deal with the loss of my mom in more of a composed fashion, plus the stress was huge associated with ensuring my dad remained okay now that he would be living on his own. Not for anything but I could swear I was limping more! Two months after my mom's passing I remember sitting down in the living room at my dad's house with my brother Anthony and telling my dad about my condition, that I had MS. I thought about not telling him so soon after my mom's passing, or even not telling him at all. But after talking it over with Luisa, my two brothers and my sister-in-law Debbie, I concluded that telling him as soon as possible was the only right thing to do. Besides, I was still feeling guilty about hiding my condition from mom and "lying" to her for several years about my limp. Not telling her that I had MS when she was alive is something that I will always regret. Should anything happen to my father and I didn't tell him, I would feel terrible and would never be able to forgive myself. This is something that I would carry with me for the rest of my life. It was time.

Telling dad was not as bad as I thought it would be, probably because he didn't really understand what MS was and probably because he was still in shock over losing my mom. I remember telling my dad that I had a mild case of MS (whatever that is), and let him know that's why I was limping. I also let him know that only my left leg was impacted, which was somewhat true. While he understood, he immediately started blaming himself much like he continued doing about my mom's death. You see, my dad was diagnosed ten years earlier with Myasthenia Gravis, another neurological condition. In his mind, he blamed himself about my having MS thinking he passed down a bad gene associated with the neurological condition. I assured my dad that MS was not a hereditary condition and that it had nothing to do with him. But in his mind, it *was* hereditary and therefore *he* was responsible. Once my dad made up his mind about something, there was no changing his thinking.

In early February 2010, I scheduled my next quarterly appointment with Dr. Blitz. My left leg had become increasingly more spastic and I was definitely limping more. We talked about my mom's passing and how stressful and upsetting it was, plus the stress associated with me now having to worry about my dad now that he was living alone. After Dr. Blitz offered her condolences, she watched and timed me as I walked. After I came back to her desk and was seated, she exerted downward pressure on my arms and legs as I pushed upward. She told me that the tightness in my left leg had not improved and may have actually gotten worse since she last saw me. She also told me that the muscles in my left leg were noticeably weaker. I told Dr. Blitz that while it could be my imagination, I seemed to be limping more since my mom died. On the Expanded Disability Status Scale (EDSS), with a zero being normal and a grade of ten signifying very severe disability or death, her assessment was that I was around a 2.5. This meant that while I did not yet have any disability, it did however show some abnormal neurological signs. Before I left her office, Dr. Blitz suggested I visit an orthopedic specialist and consider getting fitted for a foot brace which she said may ease my foot drop and may lessen my limp. I agreed, and she gave me the name of an orthopedist in the area and a script if I decided to proceed. Dr. Blitz then talked to me again about considering switching from Betaseron to Tysabri, and again told me that patients taking the drug had a slower rate of disability progression in comparison to patients using other MS therapies that were on the market. I was very honest with her and told her the PML thing scared me, so I was not really interested and it was unlikely that I would be switching to Tysabri anytime soon. At that point we dropped the subject. Dr. Blitz then told me that she would continue to monitor the spasticity in my leg and if it worsened, talk to me about other options. I was already taking six Baclofen pills per day so I knew that further increasing the medication's dosage was not really an option, unless I wanted to sleep most of the day. I got up, shook her hand and left the office. On my way out I scheduled with Donna my next quarterly check-up in May 2010 with Dr. Blitz.

Chapter 8
The Baclofen Pump

It was the first week of June 2010 when I had my next quarterly follow-up visit with Dr. Blitz. At this point, I had been fitted with and was wearing the orthotic foot brace which she had recommended for me during my last visit. The brace was made to custom fit my left foot and when I placed it inside my shoe it came up to my mid-calf. The "portable" nature of the design allowed me to use the brace when wearing any sneaker or shoe. It was made of lightweight black plastic, fit over my sock and beneath my trousers and as such was not visible to others unless I chose to wear short pants (which I did not). In years past and prior to getting the brace I would always wear short pants in the summer months, a practice that I never went back to once I started wearing it. I guess I chose not to draw attention to the brace and run the risk of people asking, "What happened to your leg?" and being placed in the uncomfortable situation of having to either lie and make up a story or go into details about my illness. Out of sight, out of mind. So, I chose to keep it out of sight and cover it up! Dr. Blitz was correct in that wearing the brace did ease my limp. It also provided me with more stability and allowed me to walk with greater speed. But even with wearing the brace and popping six Baclofen pills a day, the muscles in my lower left leg continued to be tight and would occasionally spasm. Also, bending my knee when walking was becoming more difficult. While the orthotic brace gave me more support when I walked, it also forced me to walk more stiffly. Now I know what the saying "peg-leg" means.

During my visit with Dr. Blitz she mentioned that I consider having a pump surgically implanted to administer the Baclofen. I was already taking six Baclofen pills per day, so further increasing the dosage and taking more pills each day was really not a feasible option. And even if I were to increase the dosage and take any more Baclofen pills, I would likely fall asleep at my desk in the office. Increasing the dosage would surely make me feel even more tired than I was. So I listened to what Dr. Blitz had to say. She described the Baclofen pump as being a small thin device the size of a hockey puck that is surgically implanted into the lower abdomen, and has a catheter attached which carries the medicine directly into the spinal fluid. She told me that the dosage is regulated via an external device that is waived over the stomach where the pump is implanted, and that the medicine in the pump could be replenished by her with a needle right in her office a few times a year. She told me that the refill process is quick and painless. Dr. Blitz went on to tell me that the benefit of having the pump implanted versus taking the pills is that the medication in the pump is more concentrated, goes directly into the spinal fluid and has a more immediate and targeted impact. As such, she indicated that the dosage is lower and the fatigue experienced from taking pills was generally not an issue. Dr. Blitz then told me that the procedure generally required an overnight hospital stay and is performed by a neurosurgeon that she can recommend. She gave me the name of Dr. Alon Mogilner located in Great Neck, Long Island, who I agreed to schedule a consultation appointment with. Dr. Blitz said that Dr. Mogilner would be able to talk to me more specifically about the pump, explain how it works and take me through the entire surgical implant procedure. I was genuinely excited about the thought of being able to walk without a limp and not having any more muscle tightness and spasms. I was also excited by not having to take six Baclofen pills a day and feeling tired all the time as a result.

Dr. Blitz then checked my limb movements and muscle dexterity in both my arms and legs. Next, she watched me walk up and down the hallway outside her office. When I returned back to her desk, she gave me two scripts: One for full bloodwork and the other for an MRI of the brain with and without contrast. Next, Dr. Blitz again brought up the subject of me switching to Tysabri. I shook my head no, and I'm sure by the look on my face she knew I was once again not interested in having any further discussions about it. My visit with Dr. Blitz then concluded, with her telling me to call her to get the results a few days after I took the prescribed blood tests. She also told me to let her know how I made out with my consultation with Dr. Mogilner.

The outcome of the bloodwork came back within a week and was normal. As I had to wait about a week or so for medical insurance clearance in order to have the MRI performed, it was another two weeks before I was able to schedule an actual appointment. The MRI test results came back negative, showed that there were no new lesions and that the existing lesions were consistent in size and shape with the prior examination. So far, so good. Now if I could only get rid of my limp! In the meantime I continued plugging away at my business, going to the gym about four times per week and visiting my dad most weekends. I had stopped going to PT on Saturday mornings and replaced it by attending a yoga class. The yoga thing lasted about four months, and eventually I stopped that too. While I found attending yoga each week provided me with an hour of soothing relaxation, I didn't really find it did anything to improve my MS symptoms. I had been stretching and working out at the gym anyway so the yoga stretches and moves did not really add anything new. Plus, since yoga was not covered by my health insurance, I was able to save a few bucks by stopping.

I was just getting started with my business and things were slow. So while I still remained involved with RRMS, I took a consulting position with American Express in order to make some extra money. I continued speaking almost daily with Allen and Brian by telephone, and was now physically located downtown versus RRMS' midtown location. My assignment was with American Express and was slotted to last three months; it wound up lasting eighteen months. During this time I would generally speak with Allen and Brian weekly and still maintained my status as a partner of RRMS (albeit a silent one). On an occasional weekend I would do some analysis and prepare summary narratives for one of the larger clients we were working with. I also visited with my dad almost every weekend. Each time I would see him he would go on and blame himself for my mom's death. Dad also blamed himself for my condition, although at this point he was beginning to realize after speaking with the doctor treating him for Myasthenia Gravis that heredity was not a factor in my developing MS. Still though there was a high level of stress associated with trying to grow my business, doing a consulting assignment on the side in order to generate cash, my dad's continued insistence that he was somehow responsible for my mom's death and the fact that at eighty-six year's young, he chose to remain at home and live alone. These were not the easiest things to deal with. But I persevered and moved forward, limp and all!

It wasn't until early August 2010 that I was able to schedule an appointment to see Dr. Mogilner in his Great Neck office. A middle aged and very distinguished looking man, Dr. Mogilner was extremely thorough and very personable. We spoke about my having MS and that Dr. Blitz suggested I see him. I told him about my limp, that I was experiencing tightness and spasticity in my left leg and that I was currently taking six Baclofen pills per day. "Dr. Blitz suggested I consider having a Baclofen pump surgically implanted in order to ease my spasticity and assist with walking," I said. Dr. Mogilner explained, as did Dr. Blitz that the pump consisted of a small device surgically implanted into the lower abdomen with a tiny catheter attached and routed under the skin in order to deliver the drug directly into the spinal fluid. Like Dr. Blitz, Dr. Mogilner went on to tell me that this more direct delivery method had a more immediate impact on relieving spasticity, did not cause the fatigue associated with taking Baclofen pills and was something that once implanted, did not require any further thought. Dr. Mogilner elaborated further, saying that the pump would allow the medicine to be released directly into an area of the spine called the intrathecal space and that this was a more effective way of delivering Baclofen directly into the spinal fluid. He continued by explaining that the pump is shaped like a small round disk, about one inch thick and three inches in diameter, and repeated himself again saying that the pump has a tiny flexible tube (a catheter) attached to deliver prescribed amounts of the medicine. He then described the implant and dosage change procedure. He told me that the surgery takes about forty-five minutes and usually required an overnight or perhaps two days of hospitalization, with follow-up physical therapy recommended. Afterwards an external programming device the size of a hand held calculator was used to make adjustments to the dose, rate and timing release of the medication."

"What about side-effects?" I asked.

Dr. Mogilner said that "since the drug does not circulate throughout the body and it is very concentrated, only very small doses are required in order for it to be effective. Therefore side-effects are minimal, if any at all." I asked him about the fatigue I was experiencing by taking the Baclofen pills. He assured me that having the pump installed and stopping the pills would eliminate any associated fatigue, but would not necessarily be a remedy for all fatigue I may be experiencing caused directly from the MS itself. He told me that pump refill timing depended upon the dosage and that generally people having the pumps returned to their doctor's office every three months or so for pump refills and dosage adjustments. He went on to confirm the fact that Dr. Blitz handles the refills and medication adjustments, and that this was a painless and fast process.

"How long does the pump last before it needs to be replaced?" I asked.

Dr. Mogilner told me that the pump is taken out and replaced at the end of the battery's life, which is usually five to seven years. After he was through describing specifics relating to the pump and the implant procedure, Dr. Mogilner spent about thirty minutes discussing with me my medical history and reviewing the MRI test results that I had previously sent to him at the time when I scheduled the initial consultation. He also examined the leg where I was experiencing the tightness. His goal was to make an overall assessment about me and determine whether or not I was a candidate for a Baclofen pump implant.

Toward the conclusion of my consultation with Dr. Mogilner, he suggested I consider undergoing a trial procedure to see if in fact we felt that having the pump installed was the right thing for me. He told me that the trial was done via a simple visit to his office in which Baclofen would be injected into my lower back directly into the intrathecal area. He went on to tell me that because this was only a one-time injection, the effects of the trial lasted about four to six hours and that direct injection of this concentrated dose of Baclofen would allow me to almost immediately gauge the drug's effectiveness. After a few hours the medication would wear off and Dr. Mogilner indicated I would return to my normal self. Dr. Mogilner went on to say that depending on how I felt after the trial, I could then make a decision to see if I wanted to go forward with the actual surgical implant procedure. Doing the trial sounded like a no-brainer, so I agreed to proceed and made an appointment with his receptionist to have the trial done the following week. "As long as the needle does not feel like the lumbar puncture I had done," I said. Dr. Mogilner smiled, and said it did not.

The following week, Luisa drove me to Dr. Mogilner's office in Great Neck where I had the trial done. Within ten minutes or so after getting the injection I began to notice that my left leg was feeling more limber and that I was able to bend my knee more when walking. I remained at Dr. Mogilner's office for approximately ninety minutes after the injection to be sure that it did not make my legs too loose and interfere with my ability to stand or to walk. Dr. Mogilner's assistant Maria checked in on me several times to be sure it did not, and as she put it, "develop rubber-band legs."

Maria was fantastic as she answered my questions, addressed my concerns and explained to me further about how the pump worked and what it did. Before I left, I asked Maria if she would mind providing me with names and numbers of a few MS patients that had the Baclofen pump surgically implanted that would be willing to share their experiences with me that I could contact as references. She did, and at the end of my visit she gave me a list of nearly a dozen or so patients that had the pump implanted by Dr. Mogilner. Maria told me to "feel free to call them all, or call a few at random, whatever it takes for you to become comfortable before deciding whether or not to undergo the procedure." For what it was worth, Maria was very upbeat about me having the pump implant procedure and indicated that to her knowledge and experience, the majority of MS patients who had the procedure done were extremely satisfied, with each of them feeling it made a positive difference in reducing their spasticity and improving their ability to walk. She also went on to praise the work done my Dr. Mogilner, assuring me that he was among the very best neurosurgeons around. I thanked Maria and left the office, indicating that I would be in contact with her after I spoke with a few patients to get their "take" and thought more about whether or not I wanted to undergo the procedure. As Luisa and I left the office, Maria gave us her card and encouraged us to call her if we had any questions about the procedure or any issues related to the trial.

When I arrived home later that day, I called the National Multiple Sclerosis Society's Long Island Chapter and inquired about getting some literature about Baclofen pumps. I also asked if they had names and contact information of chapter members who had the pump implanted that they could send to me, explaining that I was considering undergoing the procedure but first wanted to read more about it and speak with some folks who underwent the implant surgery. The MS Society obliged, and about one week later I received a package in the mail. I figured that by mixing up the names from the two sources (Maria's and the NMSS'), I would get a more unbiased sample of people to contact. Not that I thought Maria would "stack the deck" and give me the names of people having a strong bias toward having the pump implanted, but I wanted to be absolutely certain of all the facts and get as diverse a set of patient feedback as possible before making a final decision as to whether or not I should have the pump surgically installed. After all, this was surgery!

The literature about the pump that the MS Society sent to me pretty much described what Dr. Mogilner had told me. The MS Society also sent me the names and contact information of six individuals who had the procedure performed over the past several years who would be willing to share their experiences with me. My goal was to take at random a few names from that list, plus take a few random names from the list Maria of Dr. Mogilner's office gave me and call/email each of them. Over the next two weeks, I wound up speaking to seven people (four from the MS Society's list plus three from Dr. Mogilner's list). With the exception of one person that I contacted, everyone I spoke with said very positive things about the procedure, with each one of them indicating their spasticity was either significantly reduced or had gone away entirely. One person I spoke with said that their gait had dramatically improved by nearly 80 percent! Another three patients who had the procedure performed by Dr. Mogilner also spoke very highly of him as well, giving him nothing but praise. The one individual that I contacted who was not overly positive but somewhat neutral about the implant, and was someone who subsequently relocated from New York to Colorado, said that the pump did not really make any discernible difference compared to when she was taking the Baclofen pills. This person went on to tell me that given her experience and knowing what she now knows, if she had it to do over again she would *not* have had the procedure done.

I took a temporary reprieve from dealing with the whole MS thing and the following week, Luisa and I flew down to Florida with Lauren who was beginning college at the University of Miami. It was a short three day visit, and after setting Lauren up in her dorm we flew back to New York. I was very sad to leave Lauren behind, but both Luisa and I were confident she would eventually adjust and do well. She did not disappoint us, and her four years of college went by very quickly. The next Monday, we drove to Ithaca New York to drop Deanna off at Cornell as she began her fourth and final year of college. August 2010 was certainly a very busy and hectic month! For at least the next year, Luisa and I were alone in the house. What would we do with ourselves without having to shut off the lights in their rooms that they constantly left on or clean the dishes they would always leave in the sink?

After returning home from Ithaca, I called Maria at Dr. Mogilner's office to share some of the feedback that I gotten from patients who had undergone the Baclofen pump implant surgery. I told her that I was leaning toward having the pump implanted. Maria was very happy and said that she felt I would be making the right decision if I decided to move forward with the surgery. She also was very happy to see that I had been doing my "homework" and soliciting feedback from people who had the implant done. A few days later, I phoned Maria back and told her that I decided to go ahead and have the surgery performed to implant the Baclofen pump. She was ecstatic and said she would contact me with a date for the surgery after she obtained approval from my health insurance provider and was able to schedule the surgery with the hospital and with Dr. Mogilner. About one week later, Maria called me and said that the surgery had been approved and was scheduled for October 26, 2010 at Long Island Jewish hospital in Manhasset, Long Island. I called and spoke with Dr. Blitz to inform her of the scheduled surgery date. Like Maria from Dr. Mogilner's office, Dr. Blitz was also happy with and fully supportive of my decision to proceed.

It was early on a Tuesday morning in late October that Luisa took me to Long Island Jewish hospital in Manhasset, Long Island, for the procedure. We arrived at the hospital at 6 A.M., and we spent about an hour with the admissions team filling out papers and signing consent forms. I was clearly nervous, was somewhat hungry (after all, I followed instructions given to me and had nothing to eat or drink since 11 P.M. the night before) and was quite anxious. I think the last time I was in a hospital and had surgery was over forty years ago when I had my tonsils removed. After we were done with the admissions team, Luisa and I were asked to visit with administrators and nurses on another floor in a pre-surgical preparation area. We went upstairs and waited for less than ten minutes before we were called in. After completing a few short forms, I was asked to remove my street clothes and change into a hospital gown. At this point Luisa was requested to exit the room. We kissed one another goodbye and Luisa wished me good luck. She told me that she would be there and see me after the surgery. By now, the reality of the situation had finally set in—*I was going into surgery!*

Shortly thereafter Dr. Mogilner came by to see me in the pre-operating surgical area. He explained exactly what the procedure would entail and again emphasized that the entire surgical process would take less than one hour. He indicated that the preparation would actually take as much time or longer than the actual procedure itself would. He then told me he would be the one doing the surgery (which I assumed), and that I would be put under anesthesia and would not feel a thing (I had forgotten about the anesthesia part). I would awaken in the recovery room where I would remain under observation for about an hour like anyone does after undergoing surgery and then moved to a regular room. He asked if I had any questions, to which I replied, "No," and told him to take good care of me. He smiled and left my bed. About thirty minutes later I was wheeled into the Operating Room where Dr. Mogilner and his nurse assistant Maria stood perched over me as I waited for the surgery to begin. It was somewhat reassured to see Maria in the room. She obviously was a registered nurse and was very comforting throughout the process leading up to the procedure. She would be assisting both Dr. Mogilner with the surgery and the anesthesiologist tasked with putting me to sleep.

This was it! Before I knew it I was out cold.

The next thing I remember was waking up in recovery. As I opened my eyes, Maria was there and told me that everything went superbly! She indicated that Dr. Mogilner would be in to see me shortly and that I would be staying in recovery and moved to a regular room within the next hour or so. She went on to tell me that once the nurses got me situated into a regular room, my wife would be able to see me. As Maria was speaking with me, Dr. Mogilner came by and also told me that everything went fine. He said that once the anesthesia wore off completely within a couple of hours, the area where the pump was implanted would probably feel a little sore as would my lower back where the catheter was inserted. "That's normal," he said. He indicated that the soreness would last a few days, that I would remain in the hospital overnight and that I would likely be discharged the following day. He told me he would be notifying Dr. Blitz right after leaving me to let her know that the surgery was complete, went well and that I was doing fine. He said that after I was released from the hospital and went home, I should make an appointment to see him in his office in two weeks to have the staples removed. In the meantime, he said he would be writing me a script for two weeks of physical therapy (PT) which he recommended to all his patients who had surgery to implant intrathecal Baclofen pumps. When I asked why I needed the PT, Dr. Mogilner indicated that it would be necessary in order to help me more quickly resume an ordinary gait. As he left the room I thanked him and shook his hand. About an hour later I was transported to a regular hospital room.

Luisa was already in the room when I arrived. I told her what Dr. Mogilner said, which she already knew as he made it a point to see her right after the surgery was done to provide an update. Luisa then called and updated Dr. Blitz as well before even seeing me. Dr. Blitz told Luisa that she was going to see about having me transferred the next day to Glen Cove Hospital, a rehabilitation center that she was associated with. I was curious why I could not go home the next day and needed to instead be transferred to a rehab facility. Luisa told me that considering I would need PT, Dr. Blitz felt more comfortable having me spend a few days at the Glen Cove facility where she could periodically drop-in and see me until I was fully up and about. That sounded like a plan, so I silently obliged and did not question it. Still groggy from the anesthesia, I asked a nurse to give me some pain medication. I slept for the remainder of the day and throughout that night.

Unfortunately, I learned the next morning that there would not be availability in the Glen Cove facility until Thursday meaning that I needed to spend a second night at LIJ. "What a bummer," I thought to myself. But it really did not much matter though, as I was still in pain and was unable to get up from bed. Still in a lot of discomfort both in my lower abdomen and in my lower back where the incisions were made during the surgery, I was *unable* to get comfortable lying in bed.

I asked for more pain medication to help me cope. The medication knocked me out and I was able to sleep throughout most of the night. Twice during the evening I needed nurse assistance to get up and use the bathroom, as the pressure exerted when trying to stand on my own made the pain even worse.

The next morning (it was Thursday) I was told that a bed had become available at the Glen Cove facility and that I would be discharged from LIJ around noon. Luisa came to the hospital and helped me gather my belongings. Shortly after noontime, two members of the LIJ hospital staff wheeled me downstairs and helped me into my car that Luisa had brought around to the hospital entrance. The Glen Cove Rehabilitation facility was less than a twenty-minute drive from LIJ. When we arrived, two hospital assistants form Glen Cove greeted us, helped me into a wheelchair and took me up to a room that Dr. Blitz had reserved for me. As I was being transported, Luisa stayed behind in the admissions area filling out forms.

Glen Cove hospital and Rehabilitation Center, as far as hospitals went, was *first-class*. The facility was clean, the nurses and staff were extremely cordial and accommodating, and believe it or not, the food was pretty good too! Nonetheless, I was in a lot of discomfort and could not wait to get into a bed. When I finally got settled I asked for and was given more pain killers and slept for the good part of that afternoon. It was around 5 P.M. when I awoke as dinner was brought to me. Luisa stayed throughout the day and remained with me until after I finished eating. After continuously badgering her and telling her to leave, she finally departed around 7 P.M. and headed home. The next morning Dr. Blitz (who was the head neurologist at the Glen Cove facility), came by my bed to see me. She examined the area where the pump was implanted in my abdomen and where the incision was made in my lower back where the catheter was placed. I told her I was in a lot of pain and could not even get out of bed, since standing placed more pressure where the incisions were made thereby making the pain even more unbearable. Dr. Blitz assured me that the pain would subside over the next several days and that she would come by to see me later on that day to adjust (if necessary) the pump's medication dosage. She also told me that she would request the staff get me out of bed by the end of the week so that I could begin walking and start physical therapy. Thinking back, that first night in the Glen Cove facility was awful. I lied in bed awake throughout most of the night. I could not get comfortable. The pain was excruciating! Thank goodness for pain killers however, even though I consciously took as few of them as possible! I must say that the nurses and staff at Glen Cove hospital went out of their way to make me feel as comfortable as possible. Still though, it was a long night!

Later on the following afternoon, Dr. Blitz came by to see me again. She said that I would be getting out of bed tomorrow (Saturday) and that she would have me start physical therapy (PT) on Monday. The hospital did not provide PT on the weekends. She ordered that I receive PT for a total of five days, two sessions a day; one in the morning and one in the afternoon. In the meantime, Br. Blitz placed over my abdomen where the pump was implanted a device the size of an old Texas Instruments calculator. She increased the Baclofen dosage from the initial amount of 8 micrograms that was set by Dr. Mogilner at the time of surgery to 44 micrograms, nearly a 500 percent increase! Dr. Blitz spent another few minutes speaking with me and then left saying she was headed to the airport for a weekend conference she was attending on the West Coast. Before leaving she said that she would be back from the coast and into see me Monday morning. Long after Dr. Blitz left and I had eaten dinner, the nurses tried helping me out of bed to walk. I was feeling very wobbly (almost like I felt that time in April 2009 when I was leaving Yankee Stadium). I was still in pain and trying to stand was very difficult. Holding onto the hand rails that lined the hallway corridor outside my room, I walked only a short distance before asking the nurses to escort me back into bed. My attending nurse told me that I had enough walking for one day and that tomorrow would be another day. By this time, Luisa had come to visit me and stayed until nearly 9 P.M. After Luisa left, I was still experiencing pain but a bit less than I had during the first couple of days after the surgery. I guess Dr. Mogilner was right in saying that as each day went by, the pain would gradually subside. This time though I braved it and made it through the night without taking any of the prescribed pain medication.

Early the next morning I called the nurse to help me out of bed and go into the bathroom. As the nurse tried to get me up and out of bed, I nearly collapsed as my feet would not support my weight. I was literally unable to stand and support myself! Panicked and extremely anxious, I immediately called Dr. Blitz on her cell phone. It was very early on Saturday morning (8 A.M. in New York, and 5 A.M. in California), so I knew I would not reach Dr. Blitz right away and would have to leave a message. I left a frantic voice mail on her private cell phone, which was earmarked "for emergencies only." This was an emergency! About an hour later around 9 A.M. on the East Coast, I left Dr. Blitz a second message as I did not hear back from the earlier call I placed to her. As it was now only 6 A.M. on the West Coast and I figured she was either still asleep or just waking up. I waited another hour and as I was about to give her a third call when around 7 A.M. (California time), Dr. Blitz rang me back. I remember telling her in a panicked voice that I could not stand, that my legs felt as if they were like rubber bands and how frightened I was. "Help me," I remember saying, "HELP ME!" I remember Dr. Blitz telling me that she listened to my voice messages and knew I was distressed. She tried to comfort me and told me not to panic and that the pump's dosage was likely too high and needed to be adjusted downward. She said that she was currently in California and would be back in New York late Sunday evening and would stop by the hospital first thing Monday morning to see me and adjust the dosage downward. I was not happy with having to wait the weekend but there was little I could do except hold on until Monday. I remember reiterating to Dr. Blitz that she needed to see me first thing Monday morning. I again told her that I was scared. She further reassured me by saying that the dosage was likely set too high and promised when she saw me first thing on Monday morning that she would decrease it. She went on to tell me that I should begin to feel fine within a few hours afterwards. I told her that I understood, could not wait for her to see me on Monday and reminded her again not to forget about coming to see me first thing in the morning. I then said goodbye and hung up the phone.

The next two days were filled with anxiety. So much stuff raced through my mind, including things like: "What if reducing the dosage didn't work?" … "What if I was never able to stand and support my weight again?" … "How would I get around?" … "How would I go to work?" …"Was having the surgery a mistake?" … "What if …?" I kept asking myself if I did the right thing by having the surgery and if I should have listened to that one person I spoke with in the reference phase who was not supportive of the procedure, saying that the pump did not really make any difference and would not have done it again if she had it to do over.

Luisa stayed with me all day on both Saturday and Sunday, and did her best to console me and to try and take my mind off things. I guess after a while she got frustrated hearing me whine and complain about not being able to stand. She told me that there was nothing that could be done until Dr. Blitz saw me on Monday and that worrying endlessly was not going to change anything. Luisa was right. There was nothing I could do but wait. There was no sense in complaining. On Sunday afternoon I was further able to take my mind off things as my brother and his wife came to visit me, bringing my dad with them. Of course my dad asked how I was doing and of course I said I was doing fine. I dared not tell him what was really going on. No sense in getting him all worried and upset. After all, he just recently stopped blaming himself for my getting MS and was still taking full responsibility for my mother's death. When everyone finally left later that night, I talked for a while with my roommate Mr. Kenneth Jenks who told me some fascinating stories about his time serving in WWII. We spoke for nearly one hour and about 9 P.M., I turned in. I highly anticipated Dr. Blitz's visit the next morning.

As promised, Dr. Blitz came by to see me first thing on that Monday. It was before 8 A.M. when she came by. While at my bedside she took out her 'Texas Instruments Calculator' sized instrument and reduced the dosage in the Baclofen pump by over 50 percent (down from 44 to 20 micrograms). As she adjusted the dosage, Dr. Blitz said that by the evening around dinner time I should start seeing a difference and that by the next day (Tuesday morning), I should be fine. She told me that she would come by to see me the next day on Tuesday morning and that she already instructed the hospital staff to put off beginning my physical therapy until then. I asked her how long I needed to stay in the hospital and she told me that she wanted to see how I was doing with PT and see where things stood by the end of the week before making a decision. After Dr. Blitz left, Luisa came by to visit and stayed with me for the better part of the day. I told her that Dr. Blitz had come by very early in the morning to decrease the dosage, and I also told her what she said about my feeling better toward the end of the day and starting PT tomorrow. I spent the remainder of Monday lying in bed watching TV and reading some emails on the portable laptop Luisa had brought me. In the middle of the night I called the nurse to assist me to get out of bed so I could use the bathroom. While I was still sore and in discomfort (albeit less than before) around where the incisions were made, I did notice that I was able to stand and no longer had the "rubber-band" feeling in my legs. While I still needed the nurse's assistance walking to and from the bathroom, I was at least able to walk and stand somewhat on my own. I felt such an immense sense of relief. Dr. Blitz's words were true when she told me that "by decreasing the dosage, you will be fine." When I got back into bed, my earlier level of anxiety was gone and I was finally able to enjoy a good night's sleep.

The next morning about 7 A.M. one of the nurses came to get me up and out of bed. Her goal was to take me into the rest room and give me a sponge bath. Freshening up felt great and the fact that I was in a lot less pain than I was in a week earlier was a good thing. The nurse walked me back to bed and by now I was able to sit upright in a reclining chair, so she situated me there accordingly. As I was eating my breakfast Dr. Blitz came by and commented how much better I looked than I did just the day before. She examined my incisions, said that they were healing nicely and that by early next week would come by to remove the staples. Dr. Blitz then checked my limb movements and muscle dexterity in both legs. "Much better, excellent," she said. She told me how pleased she was with my progress and indicated that we seem to have found the right medication dosage. "Very good," she said. "I will be back to visit you Friday, but will be checking in with the nurses daily to see how you are progressing. You will start PT today and I'm sure you will find it very helpful." I thanked Dr. Blitz for her help and encouragement. She then left my room.

At 10 A.M. sharp the next day (Tuesday) a hospital attendant came to my room with a wheelchair to pick me up and take me to PT. On the same floor but at the far other end of the building, I was wheeled into my first physical therapy session where there were eight patients waiting in the "bullpen." There were several therapists there and within a few minutes each of us was assigned a dedicated person to work with for the next hour and throughout the entire PT duration while at Glen Cove. My therapist, I forget her name, was excellent! She had already been briefed on my case and quickly began to work closely with me.

Her goal was to build the strength in my left leg and help me regain a normal gait. Now that was a plan I was psyched to hear about! When my first session ended and prior to being wheeled back to my room, my therapist told me that at 2 P.M. later that afternoon I would be taken to a different area for one hour of occupational therapy.

As I was waiting for the attendant to pick me up and transport me back to my room, I asked my therapist what the difference was between physical and occupational therapy. I was told that that physical therapy tended to focus more on evaluating and improving a person's functional abilities, with the primary goal of treating movement dysfunctions (such as standing/leaning, gait, hand movements, etc.). She said that occupational therapy on the other hand, focused more on helping a person optimize their independence in accomplishing daily activities (such as bathing, dressing, bed transfers, etc.). She went on to tell me that occupational therapists also provided recommendations for suitable adaptations and the use of assistive equipment for home and office space in order to allow for a better quality of life, if necessary. Perfect! I had now completed Physical and Occupational Therapy 101 and was a resident expert in both fields!

After I was wheeled back to my room and had lunch, I was ready for therapy Round II - Occupational Therapy. At 2 P.M. I was wheeled into another therapy area, also on the complete opposite side of the building but separate from the area which I was taken to in the morning. Again, there were about eight people waiting to be assigned to a therapist. However, unlike the PT session I attended earlier that morning there were only two therapists assigned to work with the entire patient group of eight. Daily therapy activities were divided into two categories: (i) In the A.M., those that were facilitated by one assigned and dedicated therapist, and (ii) In the P.M., those (like bathing, bed transfers, etc.) that were facilitated by one therapist who was assigned to a larger group of patients.

At the end of my first day of therapy, I was exhausted. While the two separate therapy sessions did not seem like a lot of strenuous work, I guess that after having surgery, being off my feet and inactive for nearly two weeks and then being up and about, had taken its course. Throughout my stay at the Glen Cove rehabilitation center, I noticed I was fairly fatigued by the end of each day. Unlike the fatigue I experienced throughout the day each time I took my Baclofen pills, this was different in that not only did I feel tired toward the end of each day but I noticed my overall strength had diminished. I felt like I had no "oommppff." I made a mental note to mention this to Dr. Blitz if it continued. The good news was that the incision pains in my lower abdomen and back had now become just an occasional annoying ache when I moved and stretched a certain way.

Throughout the remainder of the week I attended my therapy sessions twice per day and felt my legs were starting to get a bit stronger. Luisa had visited me each day and brought with her dinner a few times. Even though the food at the Glen Cove facility was excellent, it was no comparison to Luisa's cooking. Throughout my entire stay at Glen Cove, I would speak on the telephone with both Deanna and Lauren each night as they were away at school. On Friday Dr. Blitz came to see me, checked my pump as well as the muscle tone in my legs and watched me walk. Her conclusion was that I was doing remarkably well and said she would like me to remain at the facility and complete one additional week of physical therapy. My jaw dropped! While I was disappointed to *not* be going home and told I would have to stay at the Glen Cove facility for another week, I realized that the therapy given at the facility was excellent and was helping. And besides, the Glen Cove facility was first-rate: the nurses and staff were fabulous, the food was very good, the rooms were kept very clean, the physical and occupational therapists were extraordinary and of course, since Dr. Blitz was the main neurologist there and I was her patient—I was well tended to and certainly afforded excellent care. Plus I had made a friend. My roommate, Mr. Jenks who was a ninety-one-year-old veteran of World War II. Mr. Jenks and I would talk at various times throughout the day and almost every evening after dinner. He would fascinate me with his stories about WWII, along with various stories he told about his forty-plus years of work experience as an auditor with Brown Brothers Harriman. Later that year around Christmas time, Luisa and I would pay him a visit at his home in Westbury, Long Island. Mr. Jenks - what a wonderful man!

By the next week, I was beginning to feel better and stronger each day. While I continued to have fatigue and a low energy level at the end of each day, I was beginning to notice a gradual improvement in my overall wellbeing. Luisa came to visit me each day and would bring me mail (mostly bills, which I paid electronically on the laptop computer she had brought me), newspapers and other things to help occupy my time. I remember her bringing me a book of presidential memoirs written by George W. Bush called *Decision Points* that had recently been published. When I wasn't responding to work emails, attending physical and occupational therapy, paying bills on the laptop, reading newspapers, talking with my roommate Mr. Jenks, being kept company by Luisa, talking on the telephone with the girls or taking a nap, I was able to read the 500-page book that Luisa had brought me.

I stayed in the Glen Cove rehab facility the additional week as recommended by Dr. Blitz. I continued going to physical and occupational therapy twice a day through Thursday of that week. I felt a little stronger and steadier as each day progressed. On Tuesday morning of that week Dr. Blitz came by to remove the staples. This was a painless and relatively quick process. She examined me afterwards, told me she was very happy with my progress and would recommend I be discharged at the end of the week on Friday. Dr. Blitz told me that after being discharged she wanted me to continue receiving PT at home, three times per week for four weeks. She said she would have her assistant Donna make arrangements with the rehab facility to coordinate the at-home PT visits with my insurance carrier.

Toward the end of the week, I was walking about three-hundred yards, or approximately nine hundred feet or so each way down the long hallway leading from my room to and from the PT center. In the beginning of the week I was using a walker. By the middle of the week on Wednesday I had "graduated" to using a cane. After dinner each evening I also walked about another one hundred twenty yards as I escorted Luisa to the elevator and then walked back to my room. On Friday morning Luisa came to get me from Glen Cove hospital and to take me home. Yes, I was finally going home! I said goodbye to the many nurses, physical therapists, occupational therapists and administrative staff who helped me during my two week stay at the facility. I also said goodbye and exchanged contact information with my roommate Mr. Jenks, who told me he would be going home the next day. We promised one another we would stay in touch. Luisa and I visited him at his home later that year around Christmas time. It was so great to see him! Unfortunately, Mr. Jenks passed away a few months thereafter.

Almost three weeks from when I had the surgery to implant the pump, I was finally home—just in time for Thanksgiving. Boy, did it feel good!

Chapter 9

Physical Therapy, Exercise and Staying Active

It was the week before Thanksgiving in 2010 and boy was I happy to be home. What was supposed to be a one or two day hospital stay for the pump implant surgery turned out to be an ordeal in which I was away from home for three weeks. But I was finally home and both Deanna and Lauren would be arriving in a few days from college for Thanksgiving break. (How ironic - it was exactly five years prior to this very weekend in 2005 that I experienced my first noticeable sign leading to my MS diagnosis after doing the fall clean-up and lawn vacuuming out at my house in East Hampton). I returned home from Glen Cove Hospital mid-day that Friday and spent the following weekend relaxing, watching television and reading the remainder of my book Decision Points by George W. Bush. The Glen Cove Rehabilitation center had provided me with a walker and a cane, and the nurses and therapists there told me to be careful for the first few weeks after being discharged and that I should use both devices as I deemed necessary. They also told me to have a grab-bar installed (or purchase one) for my shower, which I eventually did as a precaution to prevent me from falling. I relied exclusively on the cane after I came home and did not use the walker at all. I eventually wound up storing the walker in my attic in Jericho. It was not until four or five years later that I took it down from the attic and brought it to our home in East Hampton. Since the Hamptons house was larger and more spread out than the Jericho residence, my thinking was that down the road it may prove to be more useful there as opposed to it being stored away in the attic in Jericho. Today I seldom use the walker except when I have a bad day or when I venture out into the backyard swimming pool area of my house in East Hampton.

Later that afternoon, the Glen Cove Rehabilitation center called to let me know that the in-home physical therapy ordered by Dr. Blitz had been approved by my medical insurance carrier for four weeks/three visits per week, and that I would be hearing shortly from someone to schedule things. Literally less than two hours later, a gentleman named Dayton called me on the telephone to make arrangements to visit me at home to arrange for PT sessions. I chose Monday's, Wednesday's and Friday's in the afternoons for my hour-long PT time, with my first session scheduled for 2 P.M. the following Monday before Thanksgiving. I figured I would see how the PT sessions went before deciding to go back into the city to resume my consulting assignment at American Express. In the meantime, I was fortunate enough to be able to do some of my consulting work from home and connect remotely via computer. So the need to be physically on-site at American Express every day was not that critical.

The following Monday at 2 PM sharp Dayton the physical therapist arrived at my house. Dayton was a middle aged man with a nice disposition who brought with him a balance board, a variety of elastic stretch bands, two five pound leg weights and a large fitness ball. Trim and physically fit, it was apparent that Dayton 'walked the talk' and remained active on an ongoing basis. After all, having someone show up at your home to administer PT who was fat and frumpy was probably not the best way to promote the service and instill confidence in patients. As soon as he arrived, Dayton went right to work and had me do a number of exercises in my downstairs den with the equipment he brought. He then instructed me on how to do other exercises by utilizing my own body weight for resistance. My den downstairs would be my 'official' PT site. He left me with a number of illustrative diagrams with instructions for several exercises for me to do on my own when he was not present.

Each evening after dinner I would go back downstairs to my den and do all of the training routines that Dayton showed me, plus the ones illustrated on the papers he left for me. I would spend a little more than an hour or so each day doing the exercises and was determined to get back to 'normal' and rid myself from reliance on the cane as quickly as possible. While the therapy and exercise sessions did prove extremely helpful, they would ultimately not prove to be enough to eliminate my need to use the cane. I began to second guess my decision to undergo the pump implant surgery. After all, I never had any need for a cane before the surgery; but now I did. The second guessing quickly ended however, after my first visit with Dr. Blitz in mid-December 2010. During this visit she told me that without the pump, the spasticity in my leg would have likely increased to the point that my ability to walk could have become significantly compromised. Plus it was still a relatively short time since having the implant surgery so I knew I had to be patient and let time take its' course. I couldn't help but think the worst, and quickly began to realize that MS was indeed a progressive disease. It had been nearly five years since my formal diagnosis and the fact that I was fully ambulatory at this point was something to be thankful for, I guess. At that time, using a cane was quite dramatic for me, especially since it was an outward symbol to others that I had some type of disability. Eventually the visibility associated with using the cane forced me to 'open-up' and to share my disability with others. But for about one year, I was able to get by with telling others that I had sprained my knee or had hurt my ankle. It must have been a bad sprain that lasted a long time, as I told it to many of the same people for nearly twelve months. That lie however, could only last so long. Eventually I needed to 'come clean', at least to those people I would see frequently that would ask why I was still using a cane. Thinking back now, most people were not stupid and likely sensed something more serious existed, even though no one said a word.

At the conclusion of my visit with Dr. Blitz, she had finally convinced me after several years to switch therapies from Betaseron and try Tysabri. I reluctantly agreed, fearing PML. I guess the turning point for me came when Dr. Blitz told me that I had a greater chance getting hit and killed by a car stepping off a curb than I had from developing PML by taking Tysabri. I was also determined to rid myself from using the cane, so I was anxious to try something different. My desire to rid myself of needing a cane, together with Dr. Blitz's car analogy, further fueled my decision to move forward and try Tysabri. Dr. Blitz told me that if things went well and barring any unforeseen adverse reactions to the medication, she would only be prescribing me Tysabri for just twelve monthly infusions at which point she would prescribe a new therapy which she had not yet determined. Her rationale was simple. She told me that the longer one remained on Tysabri, the greater the risk became of developing PML. She also said that I had to be off my existing MS medication for one month before I could start taking Tysabri. I was anxious to stop using Betaseron so that I could begin the new treatment as soon as possible. During this visit I also told Dr. Blitz about my physical therapy routines, and the fact that I would be joining a new gym and signing-up with a personal trainer to help modify and oversee my workouts. I let her know that the in-home PT sessions seemed to be working out well. Dr. Blitz was very pleased. At this point the exam concluded with Dr. Blitz saying that she wanted to see me next in three months, at which time she would have me take an MRI to monitor and assess my condition.

In early January 2011 after having ended my in-home PT sessions, I returned to my consulting assignment downtown at American Express. My office was located at the World Financial Center directly across from the World Trade Center that was destroyed on September 11th, 2001. Construction of what eventually would become the Freedom Tower was ongoing throughout my assignment. I was fortunate to see the foundation laid and the structure rise substantially to nearly eighty stories before my assignment came to an end. Since I had been working remotely for a few weeks prior to returning to work, 're-entry' into the atmosphere was not as stark as it could have been. I remember my first day back to work and walking into my manager Jack Sonnenschein's office late one afternoon. I was somewhat uneasy, and came right out and proceeded to tell Jack that I had MS. I had known Jack for over twenty years. I actually began working for him in 1982 when I started my banking and finance career in NYC as an Auditor at Chase Manhattan Bank. I had always kept in contact with Jack, and doing so allowed me to keep tabs as to his whereabouts and maintain a solid relationship with him. This was a key factor that would eventually contribute to my landing a consulting assignment with him at American Express. Still though, telling Jack I had MS was not easy. I'm sure he surmised something was amiss, as the cane and the limp must have been a dead give-away. With a tear filled eye and in a broken voice, I told Jack about my condition - that I had MS. Looking down and fairly shaken I let him know that I would certainly understand if he felt it necessary to terminate my assignment. Jack laughed. He told me not to be silly. I went on to tell him that at this point my mental acuity was not impacted and that the only thing affected were the muscles in my left leg, thereby causing me to limp and walk more slowly, requiring the assistance of a cane. Jack was genuinely concerned about my health and insisted I let him know if I needed anything. He also told me not to worry about travelling, since my consulting assignment called for that. Jack said he would bring the people into NYC as necessary, or use conference calls and video conferencing where appropriate to facilitate any required meetings. As the Vice President and Head of Compliance & Ethics at American Express, Jack undoubtedly had the authority to call the shots. I remember thanking him and telling him that unless I asked, I did not want any special treatment afforded me and appreciated him not sharing my condition with others unless he felt it was in the department's or the firm's best interest to do so. He smiled and nodded and in a calm and serious manner, I remember him saying that he had no intention of terminating my contract. He went on and told me that he valued my work and that he looked forward to my contributions in the future. Jack then looked at me with a slight grin and I remember him saying: "I did not hire you to move furniture, so don't be ridiculous. Your having MS does not make any difference to me, and will in no way interfere with your contract. You're not going anywhere." Both he and I laughed. I felt a lot better, as if a weight had been lifted from my shoulders. I think Jack's line about moving furniture really helped me to put into perspective my illness and made it easier for me to tell others about my condition as time went on. It also gave me the confidence necessary to realize that having MS did not interfere or limit my abilities to use my brain power to the highest level and contribute mightily to any organization that would have me. Thank you Jack!

I guess Jack was serious when he said my having MS would not have any bearing on my assignment. What was supposed to be a three month consulting project turned into a very financially lucrative eighteen month assignment in which I usually commuted into the NYC office on Monday's, Tuesday's and Wednesday's and generally worked remotely from home on Thursday's and Friday's. On rare occasions depending on my workload, I would need to alter this schedule and go into the office more frequently. In addition, I would often do work with Brian and Allen for RRMS on the weekends thereby further contributing to my income stream. This sure beat the corporate grind, and it gave me the flexibility I initially needed to fully recuperate from my surgery!

Commuting into the city and going downtown three days per week was not always easy for me, but I was determined to do it. Had I really pushed, I may have been able to cut my face-time at American Express down to perhaps two days per week by expanding my time working remotely from home. Determined to be as active as possible and not let MS get the best of me, I continued to push ahead. I remember following my daily routine and walking to the subway one day after leaving work en-route to Penn Station to catch a Long Island Rail Road train home. As I waited for the light to change so that I could cross the street and head down into the subway, I recall seeing an Express Bus pass by with a placard reading 'To Roslyn Long Island.' I made a mental note of the bus company's name, and did a Google search of it on-line after arriving home later that evening.

I was amazed to find that a Long Island Express Bus existed and originated at a park-and-ride lot in Manhasset that was only a few miles from my house. The bus offered free Wi-Fi service and operated separate downtown and midtown routes, with the downtown bus making its last stop just two blocks away from the American Express office at the World Financial Center office where I was consulting. I wasted no time, and the next day I made the ten minute drive from my house to the park-and-ride, purchased a daily round trip ticket and boarded the Express Bus to give it a try. As far as commuting went, this was a wonderful experience. I remember the passengers being very nice and the bus drivers being extremely courteous and accommodating. I recall the drivers leaving their seats and carrying my briefcase on and off the bus. I assume that after seeing me with a cane, they knew that I would welcome any help and assistance they gave. The bus was very comfortable and not overly crowded. As it was the end of the month anyway and since my railroad ticket was due to expire, it wasn't until the following week that I changed my commuting routine for good, as it was the start of a new month. Gone were the days of going up and down subway stairs, dealing with the crowds at Penn Station to board the LIRR at rush hour and being subject to almost daily delays. And gone too were the days of having to jam into a crowded subway car en-route to the World Financial Center after de-boarding the LIRR. To boot, the Express Bus was not only much more convenient and comfortable, it was slightly less expensive than the rail road and took about the same time as my previous commute. Bottom line though, this was much easier for me! And considering I no longer needed to purchase a subway metro card, the monthly commutation savings were even greater. To this day I continue going into NYC via the Express Bus and have never looked back on my old commuting ways; I have never again used the Long Island Rail Road for my work commute into NYC. For someone struggling with MS, taking the Express Bus into Manhattan posed an ideal commuting alternative for me and was one which would only prove more palatable in the future as time would go on.

I continued to 'get out there' and be as active as I could be. In February 2011 I joined a new gym (the New York Sports Club - NYSC) and broke down and made an investment and signed-up with a personal trainer. Unlike my prior gym, this one had an elevator instead of stairs was much larger, newer and had a more expansive variety of equipment. Like my old gym, the NYSC was about two miles from my home (only in the opposite direction) so there was no excuse for me not to go. I worked out regularly and visited the gym about three times per week, plus I made an additional two visits per week to work out with my personal trainer, Chris Mills. The elevator at NYSC made it much easier for me, as I no longer had to navigate two separate flights of stairs every time I went to and came from the gym. Climbing and going up the stairs was much less of an issue when I was fresh and heading into the gym vs. walking down the stairs when I concluded my workouts and left. Going down stairs was always a bigger challenge for me anyway, and doing so after working out was at times very difficult. In addition, parking at NYSC was better as there were more parking spots that were closer to the gym.

Having a personal trainer was excellent. It forced me to focus exclusively on specific muscle groups and allowed me to tailor my individual workouts when I would go to the gym on my own. Plus it gave me the motivation I needed to continue exercising. My personal trainer Chris Mills was great, and he quickly was able to assess my condition as well as my strengths and limitations. Initially unaware of what MS was, Chris quickly educated himself about my condition and the disease itself and frequently made suggestions regarding my workout and diet. He also tailored my workouts to how I was doing on a particular day and always encouraged me to push to my limits. More than anything, Chris instilled confidence in me and would always tell me I was doing well (even on days when I knew I was not); he really helped me maintain a very positive and upbeat mindset. Chris also gave me instructions for simple exercises to do at home, which I found to be somewhat consistent with the PT routines suggested by my in-house physical therapist, Dayton. Chris also provided me with a roadmap to use when I went to the gym and exercised on my own. I continue to use Chris as my personal trainer to this day and he continues to provide me with positive feedback. He instills confidence in me, provides me with positive feedback and gives me with the motivation I need to do more.

As the year 2011 progressed, I continued commuting into the city three days per week, going to the gym, seeing my personal trainer and doing a variety of exercise routines at home. I consulted with Chris regularly and consistently researched MS on my computer at home. I became somewhat obsessed with trying a number of vitamin supplements (like Calcium, Vitamin D, Ginko Biloba, Turmeric, etc.), and tried eating several foods (like celery, nuts, flaxseeds, horseradish, etc.). I felt great and aside from relying on a cane to help me walk and wearing an orthotic foot brace, I felt as if I were at the top of my game. I was determined not to let MS win, so I frequently tried new alternative therapies including vitamin supplements and foods. In April 2011 after having a follow-up MRI done, I made an appointment to see Dr. Blitz. She was happy with my progress and told me that my surgery had healed nicely. She then made a slight adjustment to increase the dosage of my Baclofen pump. At this point she increased me to 52 mcg, a mere fraction (according to her) of the average 500 to 1,000 mcg dosage that others having intrathecal Baclofen pump implants were generally receiving. The MRI results came back and showed that my condition was stable, with no new or enhancing lesions seen. "Keep doing what you're doing" was Dr. Blitz's advice. While I was pleased I was still determined to rid myself from reliance on the cane and asked the doctor if there was anything additional I could do. Dr. Blitz mentioned that I may want to try physical therapy, which was offered on-site at the MS Center in East Meadow Long Island that she was affiliated with. I asked her for a prescription and after getting approval from my insurance company, I made it a point to attend PT twice per week. This was the second time I tried PT, and this was in addition to the excercise routines I did at the gym. I also continued seeing my personal trainer Chris an additional two times per week. Dr. Blitz also suggested that I try yoga, which I eventually did.

For the next several months, I attended PT twice a week and also attended yoga sessions every Saturday morning. By summer's end, I came to the realization that PT was not really doing anything for me and I stopped going. The exercise routines offered to me by my trainer were far more challenging, so I continued with them. By year's end I also began to realize that while very relaxing, I did not find yoga to be all that helpful in making a difference in my MS. So eventually I stopped going.

Late in the summer of 2011 I did some research and found an electronic device called the Bioness L300. The system was designed to ease foot drop by providing electrical stimulation to the foot and leg muscles. Touted as a way to regain freedom and independence by helping patients walk with greater speed, stability and confidence, the Bioness L300 was a device that could replace my orthotic foot brace. I was hopeful that it would assist me in walking better and potentially eliminate my need to use a cane. Now this sounded awesome!

Designed to help people with certain neurological conditions (including MS) walk more naturally and with increased speed and improved balance, the Binoess L300 was designed to deliver programmed, low-level electrical stimulation to activate nerves and muscles designed to lift the foot, thereby providing greater stability and improvement in one's overall gait. I was all for evaluating it and got Dr. Blitz to agree and let me try it. She wrote me a prescription for the device and I wasted no time in proceeding to order it.

I first spoke with my medical insurance carrier who told me that the Bioness L300 was deemed to be 'experimental' (even though it was approved by the FDA), and was therefore not covered by insurance. The device cost $5,200 and it seemed like a small price to pay if it lived up to its hype. Better yet, the PT area I previously had been visiting actually had a device on hand for trial so I resumed my PT visits to try-out the device and see if it worked. After a few trial PT sessions, I was pleasantly surprised to find that the Bioness L300 did give me some benefits (I thought) that were not provided from my orthotic foot brace. Looking back I often wonder if the device really did anything, or if it was all inside my head that it was really helping. Nonetheless, at the time the unit seemed to provide me with more stability and did improve my walking speed as measured by the physical therapist handling my case. Of course going through three trial sessions was not like owning the device and using it every day, but the trials were enough to convince me that the Bioness L300 was worth the investment, even if insurance would not cover it. Having an independent assessment of my walking abilities performed by my physical therapist with and without the device was the clincher; my walking speed using the Bioness L300 was slightly better!

After ordering it, the unit came to my home a few days later via UPS. I was anxious to start using it and made an appointment with the physical therapist the following Monday. After being 'fit' with the device and instructed on how to use it, I began wearing it the next day. My therapist emphasized that the unit needed to be 'broken-in' and used over a three to four week period by gradually increasing each day the time I wore it (i.e. thirty minutes on day one, forty-five minutes on day two, sixty minutes on day three, etc.), until such time that it was worn for an entire day for a ten to twelve hour period. After about one month, I was wearing the Bioness L300 for the entire day. I wore it as I commuted into the city and when I went to the gym. Still somewhat reliant on my cane, I was hopeful that over time the Bioness L300 would eliminate my needing it. Unfortunately, that was not to be.

As year-end 2011 came, I was still reliant on my cane. But I was determined not to give up. I wrote numerous appeals to my medical insurance carrier seeking reimbursement for all or part of my $5,200 investment. Unfortunately, my appeal efforts were not successful. Eventually my dad wrote me a check to cover the cost of the unit. I wore the device throughout the better part of the following year and began to slowly realize that ridding myself from using the cane was probably not going to happen. In addition, walking was becoming more challenging—even with the Bioness L300. I continued commuting into Manhattan, going to the gym and seeing Chris weekly. By August my consulting assignment at American Express ended, and I was back to working with Brian and Allen in midtown Manhattan at RRMS. Fortunately we landed a huge assignment doing discovery and expert witness work for a major NYC law firm. This kept us very busy right through the end of the third quarter of 2013. From a financial perspective, things continued to be very good!

In February 2013 I stopped using the Binoess L300 and went back to wearing the orthotic foot brace. After trying the Bioness L300 unit for the better part of eighteen months, it was becoming apparent that it was no longer helping me and that it was now time to go back and use the orthotic foot brace. I do think that the unit was helpful and that the improvements I had realized were not just a figment of my imagination. Unfortunately, it appeared that my MS was slowly progressing (even though all but one of the annual MRIs I took since first being diagnosed in 2006 showed any new or enhancing lesions). I was becoming a bit more unsteady at times. I was walking more slowly and would occasionally lose my balance. And I now needed to use a cane more than ever. Today I think back and realize that I was lucky to have started exercising, going the gym and seeing a personal trainer when I did. One thing that Chris always says to me is that he wished I had found and starting seeing him at the very beginning when I was first diagnosed with MS in 2006. Who knows, had I not started working out at the gym my disease progression may have gotten even worse. And if I started working with Chris earlier, things with my MS may have turned out differently. At this point there was no sense in me second guessing things though. I guess I'll never really know what might have been.

Later that month I went to my Orthopedist Sal, and was fitted for a new foot brace which was wider and longer than the one I had previously. I was told that the extra width and length would provide me with an increased level of support and a larger center of gravity, thereby resulting in a more stable footing that would enhance my sense of balance. He went on to say that this would thereby allow me to walk more effortlessly. Sal was correct. The new brace did just that and wearing it, along with using a cane, kept me moving. The new brace, like the old one, was inconspicuous and could be placed inside my shoe and concealed beneath my trousers. I also saw Dr. Blitz at the end of the month and explained to her how I was feeling and what was happening. I asked her why I was having more difficulties walking when in fact the MRIs I had taken over the past five or six years were basically unchanged. Dr. Blitz indicated that it was likely that my initial diagnosis of Relapsing Remitting Multiple Sclerosis (RRMS) was beginning to morph into the beginning of the secondary progressive phase. The word 'progressive' scared me, and I couldn't help but think the worst. Since I basically could not control progression of the disease, I was determined to remain as active as possible, continue exercising and keep moving.

In February 2012 I also began my next round of six monthly 'on-again/off-again' steroid treatments. I still got a temporary three or four day lift immediately after receiving the Solu-Medrol infusions. So linen closets and kitchen cupboards beware, the cleaning blitzkrieg was about to begin! I loved the feeling I got immediately after receiving the steroid infusions, and really enjoyed doing a variety of miscellaneous cleaning tasks around the house. I felt useful again, and Luisa loved that too! It's funny because in the years before being diagnosed with MS these were the exact tasks that I shied away from performing and found excuses to not do. I also enjoyed going to the gym right after receiving a steroid treatment as I felt stronger and more energetic, which typically lasted for four or five straight day's right afterwards. (Again, before being diagnosed with MS, I would find any excuse possible to avoid going to the gym and working out). I now find it very ironic how perspectives change and how not having something makes you realize how valuable the little things in life are once you lose them.

Receiving the steroid infusions often makes me think of what it is like to feel 'normal again.' This makes me momentarily wonder why this cannot be a permanent fix. Having lots of energy, maintaining an unimpaired gait and possessing pretty good balance - these are just some of the little things that you take for granted until you lose them! But I knew the reality. This fix was temporary and short lived. Making it permanent, which probably couldn't be done anyway, meant perpetual steroid use and with that would come the consequences associated with slowly destroying one's body. This was not a trade I was willing to make, as knowing the devil you know far outweighs the devil you do not know!

By the end of summer in 2012 I realized that MS was here to stay. So too was the fact that I would need a cane to walk and the realization that it was time to 'come out of the closet' and stop making excuses that I had hurt my knee. It was time to level with people close to me that I had MS. In the early days after being diagnosed, I often felt sorry for myself and silently asked "Why Me?" But I knew that the sooner I admitted to and accepted my disability, the quicker I could move on with the next phase of my life. The days of running around in college were gone. No longer was it 1979 - it was now 2012. I was no longer twenty-one years old. I was now fifty-three. It was time to face the reality that MS was here to stay, at least for a while. It was about time that I explored new ways to make the best of the situation.

Chapter 10

Using a Cane and Opening Up to Tell Others

It was the end of 2012 and I finally realized that things were going to be different going forward. I knew that my life most likely would never really be the same again, at least for the time being.

Yes, I had MS. It was time that I came to grips with it. To begin with I really had to start telling people, at least those who were fairly close to me, that I was using a cane because I had MS. I held out hopes that the pump implant, the physical therapy, the personal trainer, the various vitamin supplements, the different medications that Dr. Blitz had prescribed, the vigarous exercise programs, the Bioness L300, the yoga, etc., would eliminate the necessity for needing a cane to help me walk. I remained optimistic for nearly two years after my intrathecal Baclofen pump implant that I would be able to resume walking without assistance. But as the months passed and I became a bit more unsteady, I started walking a little slower than before and was beginning to feel much more off balance at times. I was also beginning to tire more easily, particularly on days after working out at the gym. And carrying small grocery bags from the car into the house or something simple like bringing home my dry cleaning became more of a challenge, something that used to be second nature for me. I knew that I could no longer make excuses. I particularly noticed that I was having difficulty maintaining my balance when going down stairs and walking downhill on moderate inclines. I was also having difficulty stepping off curbs to cross the street. These relatively simple routines are ones that everyone likely takes for granted, but were quite challenging for me. At times when I was struggling, I'm sure that others noticed too.

I could no longer hide from the fact that I had MS. I had run out of excuses. There was no sprained knee. There was no twisted ankle. There was no new pair of shoes that needed to be broken in, etc. MS was no longer the invisible thing that it was in 2006 when I was first diagnosed. Other than telling immediate family members, a few close friends and neighbors, my business partners and one or two other people, I had not confided in anyone else up to this point that I had MS. I imagine there were some who didn't believe the excuses I made for limping and walking with a cane anyway, and some people may have even suspected I was dealing with something more serious. But for the most part no-one ever asked anything, questioned what I said or pressed the issue. And if someone did, I would nonchalantly shrug it off and make up some excuse. Realistically though, as hard as it was to admit, I had MS and I could not hide it any longer.

I remember going alone one night in January 2013 to the wake of a close family member, the wife of my father's first cousin. Many first and second cousins, along with some distant relatives were in attendance at the funeral parlor. I navigated through the snow and ice outside in the parking lot and hobbled inside with my cane in hand. Funny because two years later in 2015, I would dare not navigate the snow and ice by myself for fear of falling. Once inside the funeral parlor at the wake, I walked up front to the coffin and paid my respects to the immediate family of the deceased. I then took a seat toward the rear of the room. After sitting there for a while, several cousins and other relatives came over to me. As we exchanged hugs and greetings, several close family members that I had not seen in quite some time saw me with a cane asked me what was wrong. For those who asked, I calmly but nervously told them individually that I had MS, was diagnosed in 2006 but was currently doing fine. I was pretty strong and direct, realizing I just needed to say that I had MS and quickly get through the conversation so I could move on like it was no big deal. After disclosing to a few family members that I had MS, I quickly changed the subject and made a conscious effort not to dwell on my condition. Inevitably though almost everyone I told initially expressed their sorrow and disbelief, and then proceeded to tell me about a close friend, neighbor or family member they knew who had MS. They quickly shared with me the various stories (some of which I preferred not hearing) of people's hardships from having the disease. It was disconcerting to hear about people in wheel chairs, people getting around on scooters, people who used walkers, people who could not maintain their balance and stand on their own, people who had trouble remembering things, people who could not see clearly out of one eye or people who would lose their grip and were unable to hold a fork to feed themselves. These were *NOT* the things I cared hearing about. I'm sure that most people thought that since my *disability* seemed fairly benign, their telling me stories of those they knew who appeared to be more severely disabled would help me feel better. After all, I did look to be in pretty good shape. While they certainly meant well and tried their best to make me feel better, the contrary was true. Hearing those kinds of stories only created more doubt and wonder in my mind about what the future progression of my MS would be. That scared me then, and it still scares me today. The good news was that by letting people talk and go on with their stories, it really took the focus away from me having to talk any further about my condition. I guess people just liked hearing themselves speak. As they told their stories, I smiled, politely listened but always did my best at an appropriate point to casually try changing the subject away from my having MS. This turned out to be good practice for me. Later on I would begin to open-up and share my condition more easily with others.

Other more distant relatives came by when I was in the funeral parlor and also asked me what was wrong. Some were discreet, pulled me aside and quietly inquired why I needed to use a cane. Others however, were less tactful and in a loud voice would say things like "Hey Vinny, getting old? What's with the cane?" I guess they forgot they were in a funeral parlor. To these people and to the other more distant relatives that I rarely saw, I would say something like: "Ah, it's a long story. I'll tell you later." What I really wanted to tell these loud obnoxious people was to go to hell and that it was not any of their business. I refrained though, and later never came. There was never a need to ever follow-up with any of them; perhaps I'll need to do so at the next wake!

Later that evening as I drove home from the funeral parlor I realized that telling people I had MS was not the big ordeal I thought it would be. All of the anticipated stress and feelings of anxiety I had leading up to my disclosure never materialized. I also began seeing that almost everyone I told knew of someone who was afflicted with MS and that they almost felt obligated to tell me about them and the challenges they were dealing with. It took me six years, but I was finally able to say it: "Yes, I have MS." There was no longer much if any crackling in my voice, nor were there any tears in my eyes or any searching for the right words. With every person I told I would think to myself—"Hey, no big deal, it's not like I'm going to be moving furniture...I need to stay focused on my *a*bilities as opposed to my *dis*abilities." And with each person I spoke to, I felt a sense of relief and really felt that I was getting stronger each time I disclosed to others that I had MS. Don't be fooled into thinking I had become a pro at saying that I suffered from MS, because I had not. It's just that the reality of the situation was finally beginning to set in after six years. The fact that I had MS became more real, and in actuality became more reinforced with each disclosure I made. Actually, I was getting fairly good at it!

As I told more people I knew that I had MS, most everyone was genuinely concerned and felt bad for me. Many times people would go out of their way to pamper me. I knew they meant well, but I was somewhat bothered at first when people treated me like some type of invalid. I often felt like my independence was being challenged. That is why in the past I tended to never let on and say anything. Common stuff that often times got to me were things like: "Let _me_ carry that bag for you," _or_ "Let _me_ drop you off in front of the restaurant," _or_ "No, you just stay home and rest—_I'll_ go to the store," _or_ "_I'll_ drive, you sit back and relax." After a while most people backed-off, but to this day there are still some who continue to coddle me. And yes, that _still_ bothers me! I guess I understand as most people really don't know what to do or say and at times and feel awkward around me. Generally though people meant well by offering to help me. To this day, I always do my best to try making everyone feel at ease and always make it a point _not_ to spotlight my disability. Admittedly though there are some days when I could use the help. Like carrying that bag, or going to the store, or dropping me off in front of that restaurant, or offering to drive, etc. As time has gone on, I've learned to ask for help when I need it most. And for the most part close neighbors, relatives and friends have learned to read me. In the earlier years after my diagnosis and even on those days when my symptoms were worse, I would always remain adamant about doing things myself and not ask for anyone's help, even when I needed it and even when help would have been most welcome. As time went on though I started asking for help when I needed it and began being honest about how I felt. I started to open up and would say things like: "Hey, I'm having a bad day, would you mind driving?" _or_ "Hey, my walking is a little off today, do you think you could drop me off in front of the store or restaurant before parking the car?"

It is interesting that my wife Luisa, who is clearly the closest person to me, continues to go out of her way and continually offers to do things for me even on those days when I would prefer to do things myself. Part of this is probably my fault as I have a long history of telling her and others that I'm feeling fine, even when I do not. Most of the time I did a lousy job of pretending I was fine; I guess the grimace on my face would give things away. And when I'm having a bad day, in addition to grimacing, I have a habit of biting down on my lip and looking down. Sometimes I make these facial expressions out of pure frustration and not necessarily because I'm having a bad day. So anyone who knows me can figure out pretty quickly that something isn't right. Anyway, I no longer try to mask the issues and hide my feelings but instead have started asking for assistance when I need it. Still though whenever I say I'm fine and feel okay, eyebrows are sometimes raised and doubts elevated at times to the point that those I am closest with do not believe me. Luisa and others still need to get used to this. It will likely still take more time to sink-in. The other part of it probably relates to the fact that since Luisa knows me best, she sees me struggling and always offers to help. I'm sure this is mostly an instinctive reaction on her part. But, I still grimace, bite my lip and look down.

As far as my interactions with others were concerned, using a cane became a dead giveaway that I had a disability. Funny because I never felt as if I were disabled at all. I remember after first telling my dad that I had MS, he told me I should get a handicap placard for my car. At first, I didn't want to even consider getting one. I could walk so I thought to myself that there was no need to get a sticker and broadcast my disability to the world. "That's for people in wheelchairs or for people who use walkers and scooters," I would tell him. Besides, I thought to myself, "there were so many other people who really needed the placard besides me; I was able to get by." Eventually I realized though that my dad was right. Having a disability placard let me park closer to my destination and made things much easier for me. As time went on, having the placard actually gave me the inducement to get out of the house and go to stores since I knew I could park close by and would not have to worry about walking a great distance across a parking lot or down the street. Also I began telling myself, "Who cares what people think?" The most upsetting thing to me was (and still is) the fact that that so many people that had disability placards on their car's looked just fine, and that more than likely I suspected that some of them may have obtained the decal by falsely making claims they were disabled. Almost always the dedicated handicap parking spots at malls or stores, which are relatively few to begin with, were taken and I often had to wait double parked until a spot opened up. As I would wait in the car for a spot I'd often say to myself, "I can't believe all these people are handicapped or disabled." And most of the time someone would come _running_ out of the store and get into their car. It didn't appear as if they had any physical disability at all, and this made me really wonder how in the world they got a disability placard. It also gave me pause to think about why I had to wait over two months and fight with Nassau County to finally get mine. And of course, there was always the occasional person who pulled into a handicap parking spot, got out of the car and walked briskly or sprinted to their destination inside the store, with no visible disability whatsoever. Unless there was something I could not see, like a mental disability, I started to think that these people were probably just inconsiderate, selfish and lazy, and that they would probably prefer not to walk any distance even though they seemed very capable of doing so. Whenever I would call them out on this (and yes, I sometimes would, contrary to my laid-back attitude to "let things slide"), I would roll-down my car window and give them a piece of my mind. Most people were usually very boisterous, arrogant and defensive—a dead giveaway that they were wrong and likely feeling guilty. To boot there was never any sign they had any type of a mental disability based on how articulate they were and the back-and-forth dialogue I would sometimes have with them. While I generally didn't let most things bother me, this one really pissed me off. It still does to this day!

As far as work went, there were many instances when my partners and I would go on various client calls and often run into and encounter industry professionals that I knew or had met during my tenure at Credit Suisse. I'd walk into a conference room where a meeting was scheduled to take place, take a seat and proceed with Allen and Brian to make our business pitch. At the end of the meetings people I previously knew, after seeing me with a cane, would inevitably pull me aside after their colleagues had left the room and inquire what was wrong. After all, in all likelihood the last time I saw them I was fine and I was not using a cane and had nothing physically wrong with me. Now when they asked I would calmly let them know about my condition and that I had MS. As far as those whom I had never met before, it was no surprise that no one ever really asked me what was wrong as they had nothing to compare with. So the subject never came up.

Everyone that I knew and who had asked about my use of a cane was professional and inquired discreetly when no-one was around. I would always nonchalantly tell them I was diagnosed with MS in 2006, began using a cane several years afterwards but that I was presently doing fine. Everyone felt bad and they all told me that I should let them know if I needed anything. I would always think to myself and wanted to say, *"Yeah, I need something—I need you to award me some business."* Of course I never did say this even though it was very tempting! I was becoming pretty good at disclosing my disability in more or less of a "matter of fact" fashion, and always did my best to quickly change the subject. Often I would do so by saying things like: "So how's your spouse doing?" *or* "How old are your kids now?" *or* "How long has it been since you started this job?" Almost every time that I looked to change the subject away from my health, the person with whom I was speaking with wouldn't let me. Instead they began to share stories with me about someone they knew who had MS. This is the same thing that happened when I told people at the wake that I had MS. As time went on though, I began realizing just how many people suffered with this horrible disease.

Another thing that I began to discover as I disclosed to others that had MS, in addition to learning that so many other people also had the disease was that countless others had medical conditions seemingly a lot worse than mine. As I opened up to those close to me and told them I had MS, their initial response was to say, "I'm sorry." Some of them would go on and tell me about someone close to them who was diagnosed with a potentially fatal disease. A condition like stage 4 lung cancer, or someone who had a stroke and was unable to speak or walk, or someone who was hit head-on in a car by a drunk driver who survived but was now a quadriplegic. Wow! I guess that when I told people I had MS they felt somewhat uncomfortable and many of them instinctively starting telling me stories about others with seemingly far worse conditions. I imagined this allowed them to casually move the subject away from my revelation. Or perhaps they thought that telling such stories would make me feel better. I also assumed that by them sharing their stories with me about others, it helped them feel more comfortable and at ease chatting with me after I disclosed my disability.

One story that really stuck with me though was when someone told me about a close friend of theirs, a forty-year-old woman they knew that completely lost sight in both eyes after being diagnosed with a rare viral infection (no, it wasn't MS). The person went on to tell me that while her doctors were able to successfully treat and "cure" the virus, the woman's vision in both eyes was lost for good. I again double checked and verified with the person telling me that their close friend did _not_ have MS! After suffering and being kept in the dark (literally) for six months about what was wrong and what her final fate would be, her doctors shared the reality with her that she would never see again. "Wow," I thought to myself, "people really do have things wrong with them that are a lot worse than my having MS." Putting things into perspective and if I had a choice, I'm pretty sure I would rather have my vision and *not* have to go through the rest of my life as a blind person versus having Multiple Sclerosis. I guess everything is relative though. It was at this point that I began being realistic with myself and started thinking that things could be a lot worse. "Why *not* me?" versus "Why me?" became a more common question that I began to ask myself.

There were also a few occasions for my business that I would travel with my partners to attend industry conferences or seminars. Here I would frequently run into people I knew and did not see very often. Most of the time these people would see me limping or walking with a cane and ask why. I made it a point that unless I knew the person fairly well and planned on seeing them regularly in the future with some degree of frequency, I would use the standard line of "It's a long story, I'll tell you later." Once or twice people would be persistent with their questioning. Whenever that happened I would generally stick to my guns and would not disclose my disability to those people I did not really know that well. The majority of the time however, the question never came up again and the issue just died. Whenever I would travel, my business partners Allen and Brian were great. They would always assist me—whether it be at an airport, in a hotel, at a restaurant, in a conference center or at a client's office. At times I felt like a nuisance. But both Allen and Brian told me I was not being bothersome and assured me repeatedly that it was their pleasure to help me. They confided in me that they were not sure how I was able to do it, and often times gave me high accolades for getting around and would call me a "trooper." I'd smile whenever they would say something like this. Inside, this made me feel really good.

On one trip the three of us travelled to Dallas Texas to attend the annual Mortgage Bankers Association (MBA) convention. At the convention we had a display booth that would allow us to meet with several hundred attendees over a three day period. The booth was strategically positioned in a "high traffic" area near the entrance to the convention hall. We had numerous promotional display items, giveaways and handouts available at our booth as well as a table with three chairs. Over that upcoming three-day period, getting up and down from sitting at the table to greet and speak with people stopping by our booth was *not* something I was looking forward to doing. Nor was this something I was even sure that I could do. Realizing this and without me even asking, both Allen and Brian scoured the huge hall before the convention began on day one and found (*"borrowed"*) a high stool that would allow me to remain seated as I greeted and spoke with guests that stopped by the booth. More importantly this high stool allowed me to maintain eye-level contact with guests who stopped by our kiosk without me having to leave my seat.

Maintaining eye-level contact with each attendee without having to stand up and sit down—wow, what a godsend!

I placed my cane under the table, and over the course of the next three days virtually forgot about it, using it only occasionally whenever I needed to visit the restroom. Allen and Brian made it a point to bring me lunch each day from the buffet that was set up at the far end of the convention hall so there was no need for me to get up for food. Early each morning we would arrive a little early before the exhibitors so we could walk (in my case, hobble) up and down each aisle in the conference hall to get a feel for the companies in attendance. And oh yes, we'd help ourselves to the free "giveaways" (like flash drives, stress balls, etc.) that the different vendors had on display. In the mornings and in the evenings we would eat breakfast and dinner in either the hotel or in a nearby restaurant. It was at this point in time that I needed to break out the cane! Using it was now beginning to feel more natural (although having to use it *still* sucked)!

When I would commute to and from New York City for work on Mondays, Tuesdays and Wednesdays I would usually board the Express Bus at a similar time each morning and evening. As such, I would regularly see the same people each day. For a long time I had never disclosed my disability to any of them. No one ever asked, but almost daily there were a few of the same people I would see that insisted on carrying my roller briefcase on and off the bus. They would see me each day limping onto and off the bus with my cane and always went out of their way to help. It wasn't until about two years had gone by that I shared with one or two people that I had MS. Like those people I told in the past, their reactions were similar. They felt bad, told me stories of those they knew who had MS and even shared with me stories of people they knew who seemingly had more severe ailments and conditions than mine. As far as the bus drivers were concerned they may have surmised there was an issue based on my limp and my use of a cane, but I never personally disclosed anything to them about my having MS. And, they never asked. Nonetheless the drivers always went out of their way to help me board and de-board the bus. They were always courteous and conducted themselves in a very professional manner. Who knows, perhaps one or two of my fellow commuters shared with them at some point that I suffered from MS. I would be sure to take good care of the bus drivers with an envelope around holiday time.

One day at work I had a discussion with our chief legal counsel, Brian Bluver and disclosed my disability to him. As I worked closely with Brian every day, I thought it only fair that I be upfront with him. In his mid-thirties, Brian was a very fit looking young man who always went out of his way to help and look after me. Whether it be offering to walk downstairs to buy me soup to eat at lunch with the sandwich that I brought from home, or cautioning me as I left each evening to be careful walking when there was any inclement weather, or offering to heat-up in the microwave food I brought for lunch, etc., Brian was always there for me. He would see me limp each day but never inquired why, even though I'm sure he was curious and wanted to know. Like most people I would encounter, Brian would never succumb to his own curiosity and ask. Instead I assumed he knew that something was amiss and figured that if I wanted to, I would disclose things to him in due time. He was right.

I remember talking and sharing my condition with Brian one day. I was somewhat surprised when after we spoke, he informed me that over twenty years ago he underwent a heart transplant. Brian went on to tell me that when he was about ten years old he was hospitalized with a severe heart ailment and that his only chance of survival depended on him receiving a new heart. At the time, Brian was about forty-eight hours away from death. Fortunately, a matching donor heart was identified at literally the eleventh hour. At a very young age, Brian was rushed into surgery and underwent a heart transplant. This is something that less than fifty years earlier was virtually unheard of in real life. His story really made me stop and think, and it reminded me just how bad things could be. Brian was indeed a fighter and had a very positive attitude. "Why *not* me?" took on new meaning and I realized how fortunate I was. While having MS was certainly no walk in the park, it certainly was not the worst card hand that I could be dealt. Brian likely knew the frustrations that I was feeling and what I was going through, and always showed compassion and understanding. He continues to do so. After hearing his story, I developed a different perspective about Brian and would go out of my way to help him whenever I could. It's interesting how hearing about other people's mortality makes you step back, stop and think and really appreciate what you have. It also makes you go out of your way to help them!

As time went on and I became more comfortable talking about my condition, I found myself more frequently conversing with others about the fact that I had MS. It wasn't until 2013, seven years after my initial diagnosis that I was able to tell others unemotionally that I suffered from MS. When doing my daily activities, whether it be commuting into the city for work, going to the gym, going grocery shopping, attending a concert or sporting event or doing one of my infamous "Target runs," I adopted the attitude that I really did not care what others thought about me limping and at times struggling when performing daily day tasks. On occasion people would stop and ask me, "What's wrong, can I help you?" And unlike the previous responses I had used for nearly seven years after I was diagnosed (when I did all that I could to avoid responding honestly whenever I was asked what was wrong), I would now share my story with others. Back then I would respond by simply fabricating a story and telling others something like I had sprained my knee or hurt my leg, etc. Today, I have no issues saying that "I have MS, and sometimes have trouble walking and keeping my balance." I no longer get choked up and hesitate to say I have the disease. Surely I do not make it a point to share my illness with just anyone and will generally only disclose my condition to people I know fairly well. I'm not proud to hold the MS Banner, but I am no longer ashamed either to say that I have MS.

My comfort speaking to others close to me about my condition has truly been genuine. Lately I no longer avoid or change the subject when acquaintances or those people I don't know very well ask me, "What's wrong?" I recall once at the gym a middle-aged man, who tremored slightly, approached me and politely asked in a slurred and slow speech pattern if I minded if he asked me something. "I have seen you here [at the gym] at least twice a week for several months now, with your cane. May I ask what your issue is?" He went on and quickly apologized to me for asking. He then told me that it was okay if I did not want to answer

160

the question and if I preferred to tell him to go away. I immediately said, "No, I don't mind at all you asking. I have MS, and was diagnosed with it in 2006." I went on to tell him a bit more about my disability and then said that I believed it important to exercise regularly and that I had actually joined a gym a few months before being formally diagnosed. I told him that I was determined to remain as active as possible so that I would be fit and ready for when the "cure" comes about in a few years. "That's why you see me here so often," I told him. "Great attitude," he said. He went on to tell me that he too had a neurological condition. He told me that he was diagnosed with Parkinson's disease in 1998. "That's why I shake [and] speak slowly and slur my words. I only started going to the gym less than a year ago and I wish I had joined like you when I was first diagnosed," he told me. We chatted briefly and we then shook hands, wished each other luck and finished our workouts. I did see him on occasion at the gym a few more times, but only for the next six months or so. Since the end of 2013 I never did see him at the gym again.

It was so easy and natural for me to tell this man whom I had never met before that I had MS. Had I met him a year or two prior, I probably would have taken him up on his offer to not answer his question and refrained from discussing my issue. More than likely I would have either changed the subject or just walked way. I certainly would have shied away from discussing my issue in detail with him and would have been ashamed to disclose my disability.

It took me a while but now I now know that MS is a permanent fixture in my life. This is at least the case for the time being. It is a fact that I am no longer ashamed of. I have taken on the attitude of "Who cares what people think?" I now channel my energies more positively into caring for myself and knowing that I have MS versus caring about what others may think about my having the condition. This in the long run has proven to be a very beneficial attitude that continues to serve me well.

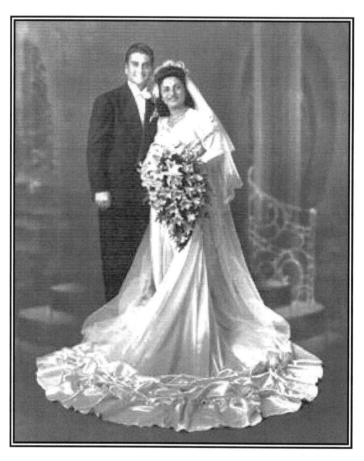

July 26, 1947: My mom (Rosalie Spoto) and dad (Joseph Spoto) on their wedding day.

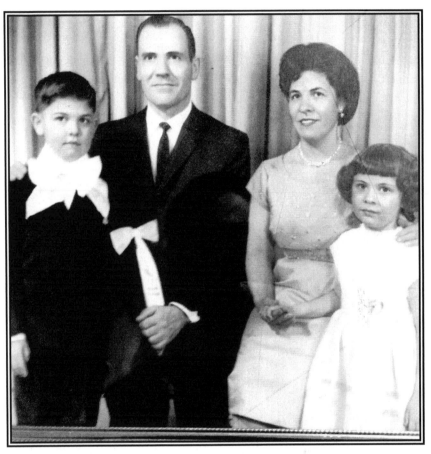

Luisa's family, circa 1962: Left to right - my brother-in-law (Anthony Conte) on his communion day, with my father-in-law, (Mario Conte), my mother-in-law (Angelina Conte), and my wife (Luisa).

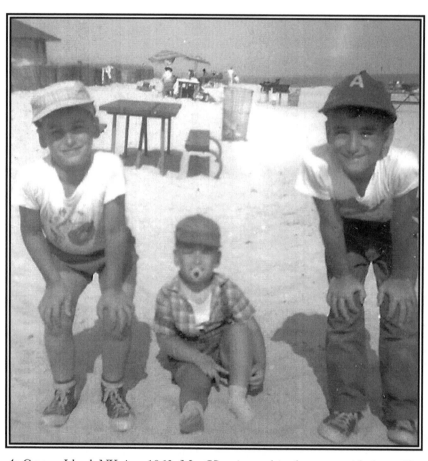

At Captree Island, NY circa 1963: Me, (Vinny) seated in the center with the pacifier, along with my two brothers - Angelo (to my left), and Anthony (to my right). Even if I wanted to, hiding my "heritage" would be impossible; true "good-fellas" - I guess!

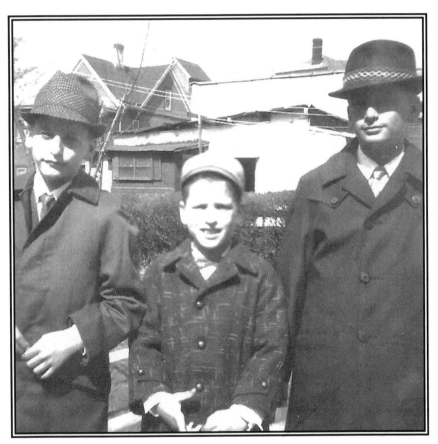

Wearing our Sunday best: Me (Center), with my two brothers - Anthony (left) and Angelo (right), in the backyard of our house in Richmond Hill, Queens NY, waiting for our parents before going to church on a Sunday morning in the spring of 1965. Check out those hats!

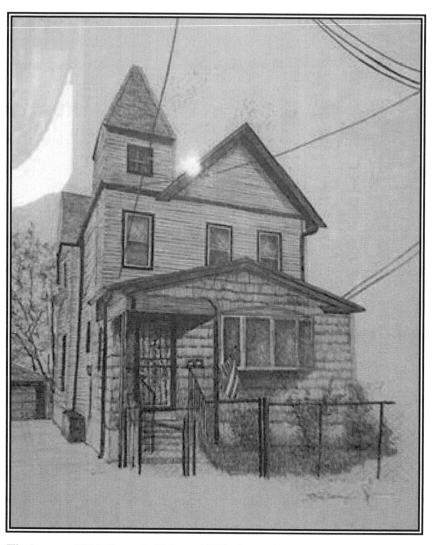

The house on 107th Street in Richmond Hill, Queens New York that I was born and raised in.

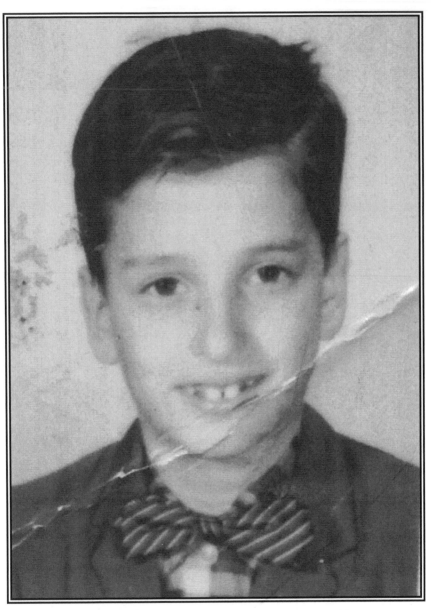

Class picture - Me, 1st grade. What a handsome dude (Not)!

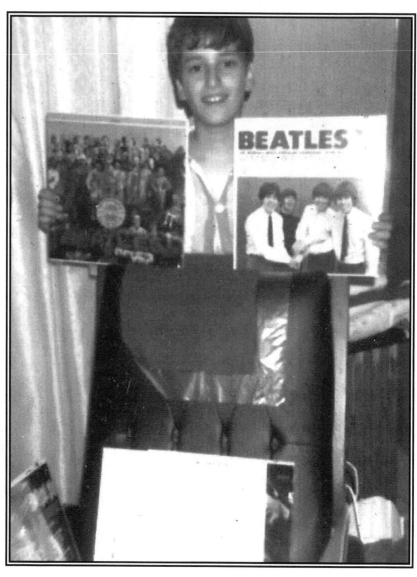

Christmas morning, 1968: Me waking-up to find under the Christmas tree every Beatles album that had been released to date.

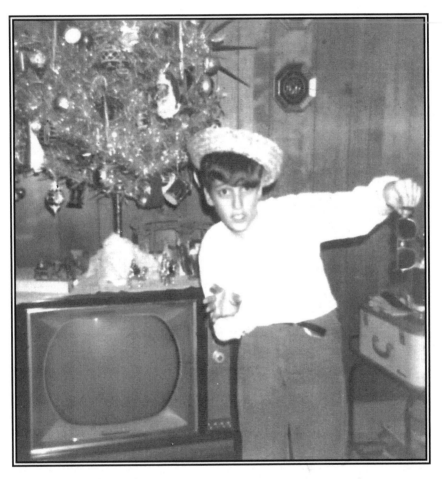

Christmas time, 1969: Me being cool - notice the artificial "aluminum" Christmas tree behind me and the black-and-white console television (big channel selector and all) - there was no remote control back then!

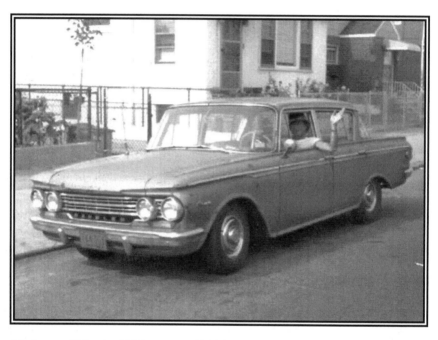

My 1st car: Taken in 1976, a 1962 AMC Rambler handed down to me from my father when I first received my driver's license and turned 17. Back then, the car's push-button transmission and reclining bench seat was a true novelty. No, this picture was not taken in Cuba!

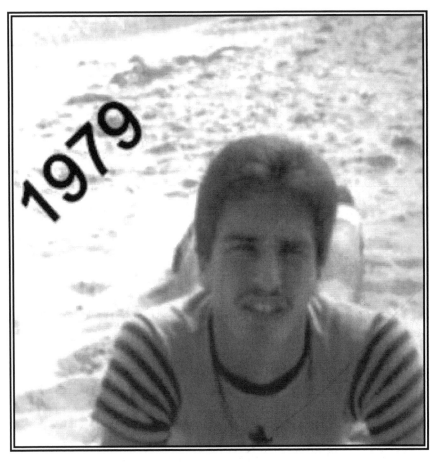

Chilin' on the beach: Me in July, 1979 relaxing at Ponquogue Beach in Hampton Bays, Long Island, NY - without a care in the world. Ahh, to be twenty years old again!

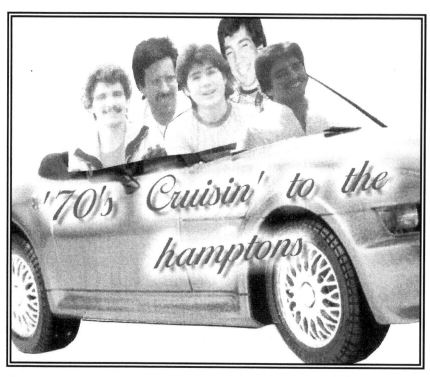

The "Hamptons Classic" crew: July 1979, from left to right - Jerry Passaro, Mike Delio, Nick Vissichelli, Rob De Tullio and Me. For two summers (1979 and 1980), we made the Hamptons our weekend home hitting the beach during the day, doing happy hour at the Boardy Barn in the afternoons, going to bars & clubs in the evenings and stopping at the Hampton Bays Diner for our usual late night Saturday 4AM breakfast - what a routine!

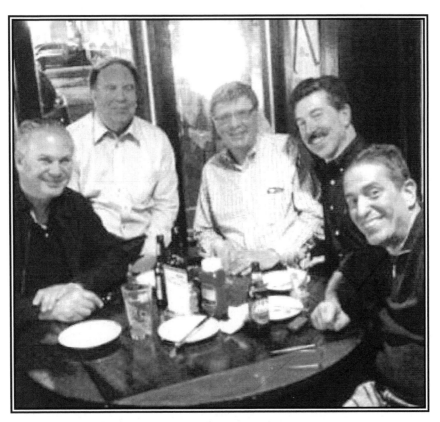

2014, from left to right - Nick Vissichelli, Mike Delio, Jerry Passaro, Rob De Tullio and your's truly. Unlike 1979 when we could stay out all night, nowadays we all have to be home no later than 11PM in order to take our medications!

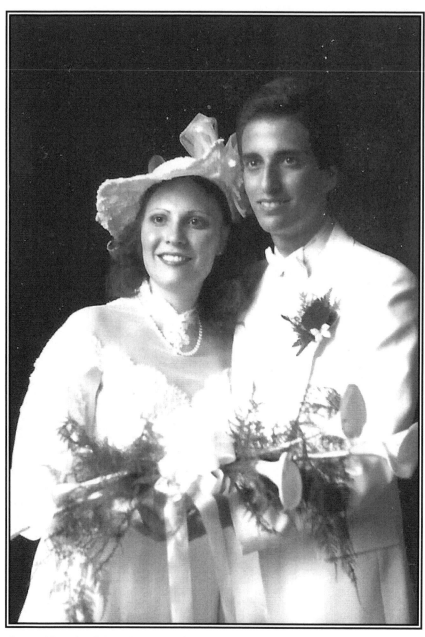

Our wedding day: Me and my beautiful bride, Luisa Conte Spoto - June 30, 1984. Boy, did it rain that day!

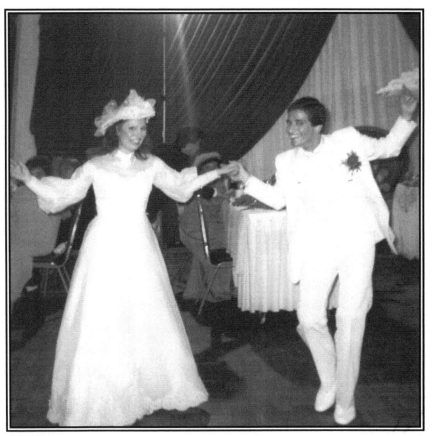

"Cutting the rug" with my wife Luisa back on our wedding day in 1984: Nowadays, I need a knife and a pair of scissors in order to cut a rug!

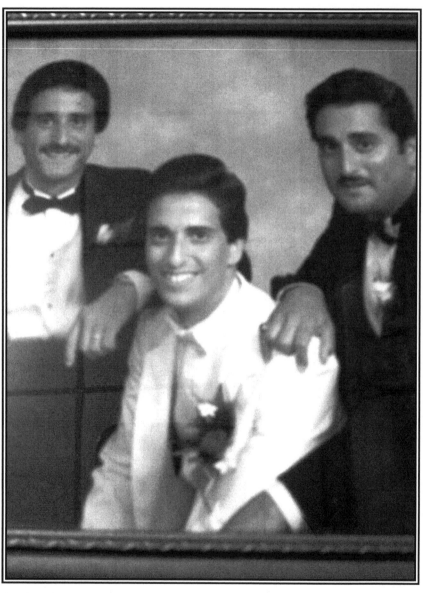

The "three amigos" on my wedding day in 1984: Me (center), and my two brothers -
Anthony (left) and Angelo (right).

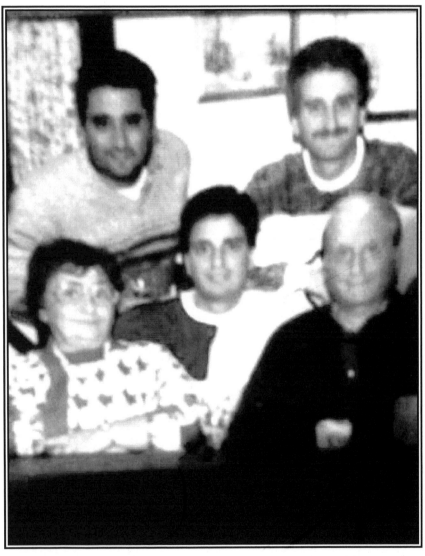

Christmas dinner in 1987: Me (center) with my two brothers (Angelo - top left, and Anthony – top right), my mother Rosalie (bottom left) and my father Joseph (bottom right).

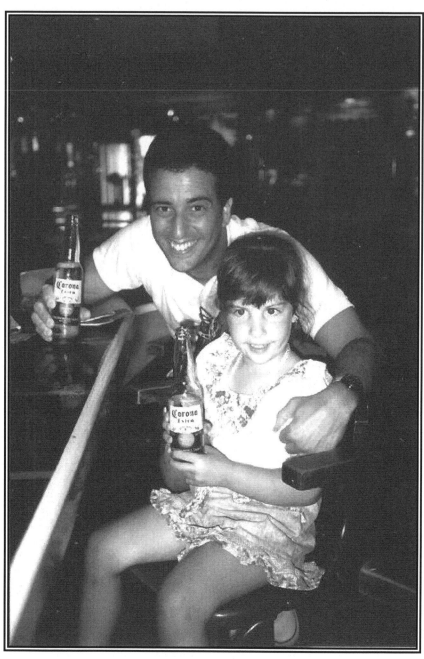

South of the border: Your's truly, with my daughter Deanna enjoying a "cold one" while on vacation in San Diego, California (August, 1991) - taking a day trip south of the border to the Hard Rock Café in Tijuana, Mexico.

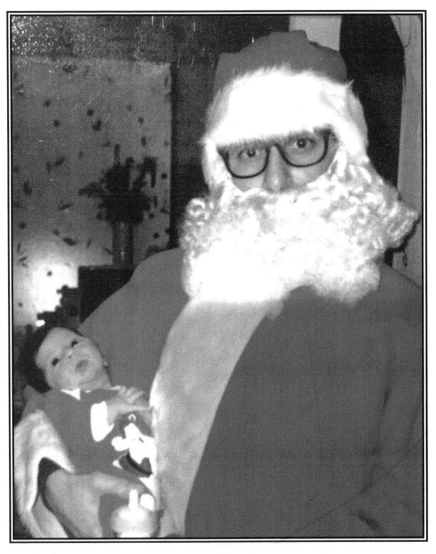

Christmas Eve, 1991: "Santa Claus" - (look at those glasses), with my daughter Lauren who we just brought home from the hospital after she was born three days earlier. Thank you Santa!

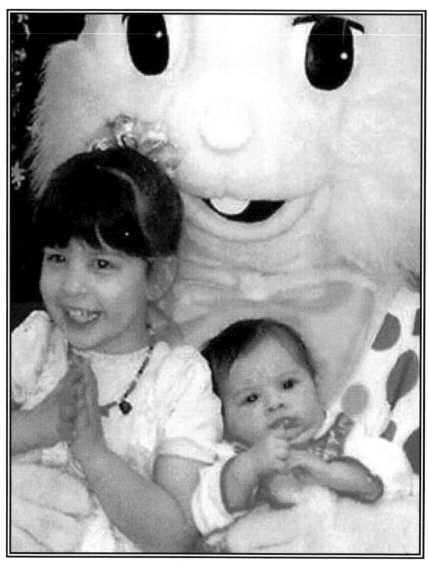

Easter: My two daughters visiting the Easter Bunny in April 1992 - Deanna (left, age 3), Lauren (right, 5 months) and the Easter Bunny (center, age unknown).

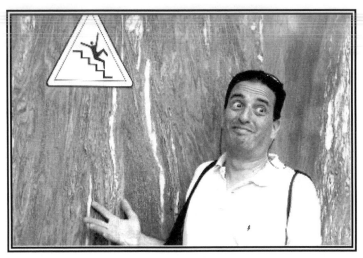

Vacationing in Italy: On vacation in Rome, Italy in August 2004. Me, clowning around and posing for a picture pretending to be falling down a long set of curvy winding stairs at the Vatican in front of a placard signifying a person running and falling. Luisa, Deanna and Lauren all insisted I pose for this picture in front of the sign, signifying my clumsy ways. Who knew?

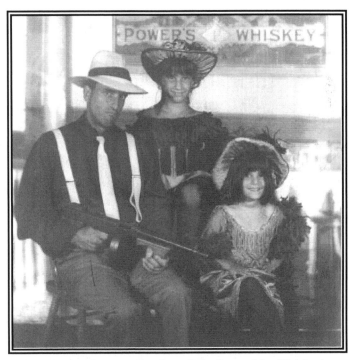

My first 'solo' vacation with my two daughters: Lake George, New York in August, 1996 - Me (left), Deanna (center, age 8) and Lauren (right, age 5). Luisa, while happy I was spending time with the girls, was not happy that I was venturing out solo for 3 days - just me and the girls. I'm sure though it gave her a welcome and much needed break.

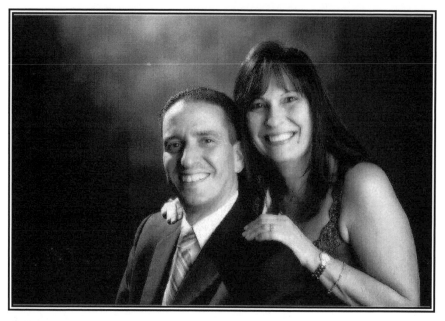

July/August 2006: Me and Luisa, taken right around the time that I was diagnosed with MS.

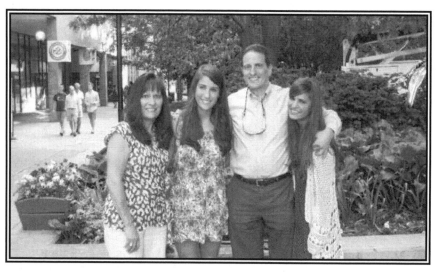

Deanna's undergraduate Graduation from Cornell University, May 2011: From left to right - Luisa, Deanna, Me (the proud "papa") and Lauren.

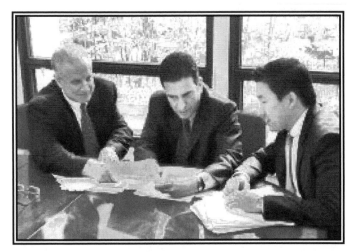

Hard at work in 2012: Me (center) with my two business partners - Allen Gutterman (far left) and Brian Lin (far right).

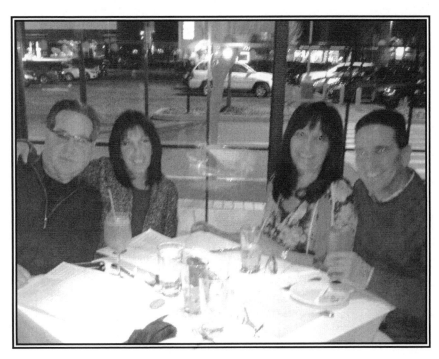

New Year's Eve, 12/31/13: Out to dinner celebrating New Year's with our neighbors (from left to right) - Jerry Roscwalb, Leslie Roscwhalb, Luisa Spoto and yours truly.

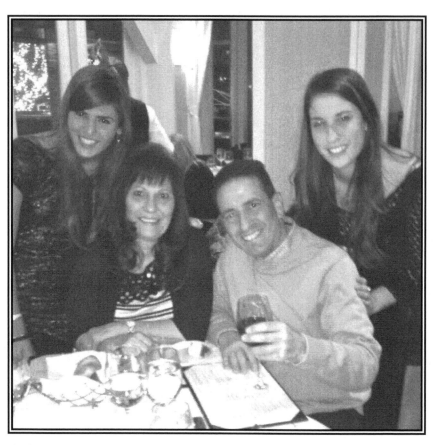

At dinner celebrating my daughter Lauren's 21st birthday on 12/20/12: From left to right - Lauren, Luisa, Me and Deanna.

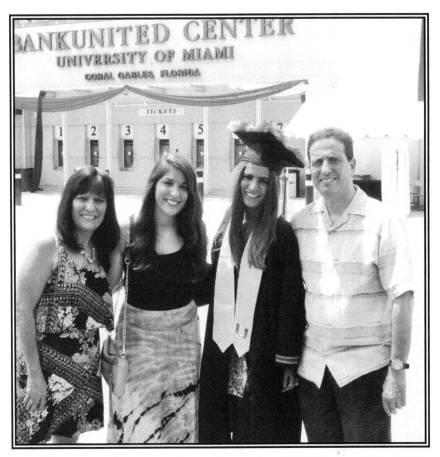

My daughter Lauren's undergraduate graduation from the University of Miami, May 2014: From left to right: Luisa, Deanna, Lauren and Me (once again, the proud "papa").

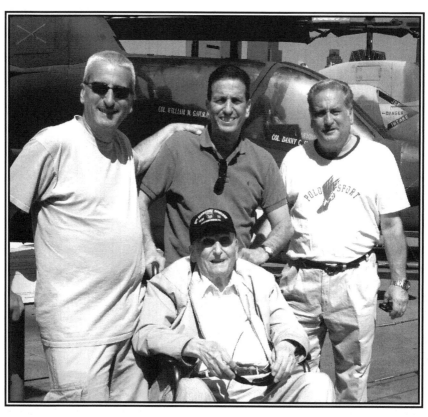

Visiting the USS Intrepid in July 2014: With my dad Joseph, who had turned 90 one month earlier (in the forefront), my brother Anthony (standing, left), Me (standing center) and my brother Angelo (standing right). This was dad's first visit back to the Intrepid in over 65 years, when he returned home on it from the Philippines in 1945 at the end of World War II. He was so proud, especially when he was asked by two out-of-town tourists for his autograph!

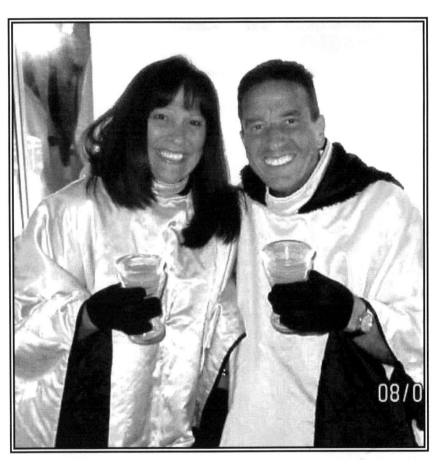

Vacation, August 2014: Luisa and I on a cruise to Bermuda, celebrating our 30th wedding anniversary.

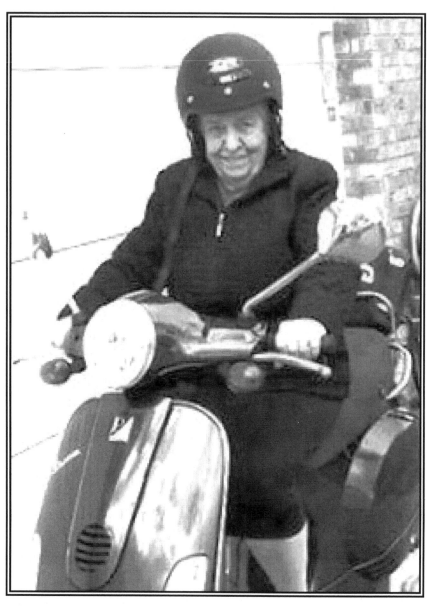

March, 2015: My mother-in law Angelina Conte "feeling her oats" at age 87, getting ready to hit the fruit store in Howard Beach, Queens NY on my brother-in-law Tony's Vespa.

Chapter 11

Changing Medications, Starting Tysabri and Exploring
Complimentary Alternative Medicines and Therapies

I reluctantly agreed to try Tysabri at the end of 2010 at the suggestion of Dr. Blitz. The thought of contracting PML really frightened me. This was despite the fact that I knew there was such a remote chance of me contracting it. At one point I even took the special blood test to determine if I had the antibody for the John Cunningham virus (known more commonly as the JC virus). If I did have it, there would be a greater risk of me contracting PML as compared to a person that was taking Tysabri and who tested negative for the virus. Sure enough the test results actually came back positive and after over one year of thinking about switching therapies, doing a lot of research, conducting countless google searches and hearing my neurologist talk positively about me switching to Tysabri nearly each time I visited with her, I decided to give it a try. This was despite the fact that I tested positive for the JC virus. To put it mildly, Dr. Blitz was very pleased with my decision. But having tested positive for the JC virus and therefore being at a greater risk for potentially contracting PML I knew that making the decision to try Tysabri was somewhat counter-intuitive and went against common logic. All things considered and after much thought and self-reflection, I made the decision to move forward with the drug and take the *very* remote PML risk in hopes that Tysabri would be the "silver-bullet" that may eradicate my MS symptoms. (Thinking back now, I cannot believe I went forward and made the decision to try Tysabri, especially considering the risk of possibly developing a life-threatening disability associated with the brain which was often times fatal). I guess as you get older you become more risk averse; time to try my luck in Las Vegas!

Dr. Blitz had previously told me that she only wanted me to be on Tysabri for twelve months, as apparently there was evidence to indicate that the risk of developing PML could increase with prolonged use of the drug beyond one year. This was an even more important fact since I tested JC positive. After I would have completed my twelfth infusion, Dr. Blitz said she would reevaluate my condition and recommend another treatment option for me at that time. For the time being though she wanted me to begin treatment as soon as possible after I had been off my current medication, Betaseron for at least one month. So I "packed my bags" (figuratively) and took a one-month drug holiday. Something to look forward to I guess.

After I made the decision to start Tysabri, it seemed like the floodgates opened up. I was barraged with all kinds of disclosures and asked to sign what seemed like an endless number of consent forms. I read through everything and signed each form that I was asked to. I scheduled my first infusion for the middle of the following month, in January 2011. Given the direct and often times very harsh warnings I was given and asked to acknowledge receipt of, I often wondered how and why the Food and Drug Administration could have approved this medicine for use. This makes me think about all those various medications advertised on television where the drug's side-effects are extensively discussed and seem far worse than the ailment being targeted for treatment.

Unlike the previous medications I had been on, Tysabri came with a "boxed warning." In addition, all of the drugs I had been on previously were administered via self-injection either weekly, daily or every other day. Tysabri was administered differently—given by infusion once per month for about four to six hours and only done at authorized infusion centers with qualified nursing staff on hand. The good news was that there would no longer be a need to worry about administering daily, every other day or weekly injections. Tysabri offered "one-stop-shopping" in that I only would only need to take the medicine once per month and no longer had to worry about forgetting to give myself an injection. Plus, traveling (not that I was doing much of it anyway at this point in time) would be so much easier too as going through airport security with needles and syringes and explaining my case to some random TSA Agent was now a thing of the past.

The infusion center I chose was in Plainview, Long Island, and was only a few miles from my home, so traveling there was not a big deal. Once there the actual infusion took approximately three hours. There were also defined points throughout the process whereby the infusion drip would be stopped for a check of my pulse, blood pressure and other vital signs. In addition, there was a post infusion observation period which lasted approximately one hour. All in all, I would be at the infusion center for over half a day, or about six hours. When I was about to begin treatment I thought to myself that this drug must really be powerful and effective given all the preparation, warnings, disclosures, vital-sign checks and observations that took place. I remember my first Tysabri infusion and how I barely slept the night before. I was nervous, quite anxious and unsure what to expect. Would I get a headache? Would I tolerate the drug well? Would I get an allergic reaction? Would it hurt? What about PML? Luckily, Luisa accompanied me on my first Tysabri infusion visit to lend support and ease my fears.

191

Other than hearing the words Progressive Multifocal Leukoencephalopathy (PML) used dozens of times throughout the initial infusion event (I initially could not even pronounce what PML stood for, but I eventually very quickly became highly proficient at what it meant and how to say it), my first Tysabri infusion itself went quite well and was not really all that remarkable. During and after the infusion, there were no headaches (which was what the administering nurse seemed most concerned with), no dramatic spikes or decreases in my blood pressure or pulse, no rashes, no allergic reactions, no pain. Nothing. All my worrying and anticipation was for naught. I was able to sit back and relax in a big reclining chair, read, watch television and occasionally grab a cat-nap or two. I even remember being on a work-related conference call for a couple of hours during one of the infusions. Of course, I had visions of being able to run a marathon when I was all done; sadly, that did not happen. Leading up to first infusion, I probably spent the course of nearly one week (elapsed time, of course) researching Tysabri and trying to find out how it worked and if proved helpful to those taking it. Of course like anything you see and read on the internet, there was a large number of varied patient testimonials. These ranged from "I saw no difference" to "It's the greatest thing since sliced bread." I was waiting for a testimonial that said it started your car remotely and changed your motor oil too! To that end, a few patient testimonials I read and video clips that I watched had people suffering from MS talk about how Tysabri transformed their lives and how it had allowed them to resume near normal activities. I remember one woman who said she was an avid jogger and gardener prior to being told she had MS, who then had to stop doing these activities one year or so after being diagnosed. She claimed that within four months of taking Tysabri, she was able to resume jogging three times per week and gardening on the weekends. "Good for her," I thought, "I should only be so fortunate." Other testimonials were less dynamic and animated and did not reveal much if any real positive changes to patient disabilities. Still though, I went into the first infusion feeling very nervous but at the same time feeling quite enthusiastic and optimistic that this new therapy, Tysabri, would help transform my life. Like I was each time I began taking a new drug or started taking a new vitamin supplement or tried a new complimentary or alternative therapy or treatment, I was excited. I was truly hopeful and kept a positive attitude by telling myself, "This is the one!"

After completing the first treatment I remained cautiously optimistic that I would see a positive change. This was despite the fact that my neurologist emphasized that the drug's purpose was not to cure the disease or completely eliminate its symptoms, but instead to halt or significantly stop disease progression. Dr. Blitz did her best to manage my expectations. Still though I was excited and remained hopeful. After a few days passed from my initial infusion and things remained relatively status quo, I convinced myself that since this was only my first treatment I had to wait a while and undergo a few more monthly infusions before I would experience any positive changes. After receiving the second infusion in February, there was no change in my condition. After the March infusion, no change. After the fourth infusion in April 2011, I felt more or less the same as before I started my treatment with Tysabri. I began to realize that I may not actually see any positive changes at all from the drug and that Dr. Blitz was probably right. Still though I continued taking my monthly infusions of Tysabri for the remainder of the year as prescribed, until the twelfth and final one was administered in January, 2012. Throughout the entire process, I remained very positive and hopeful. As the infusions turned out to be no big deal, Luisa accompanied me only for the initial one (I think). After that, I flew solo.

It was January 2012 and I had done my twelfth and final Tysabri infusion. It was now time to have another MRI done and talk with

Dr. Blitz about starting a new drug treatment. As in the past, findings from this MRI were consistent with ones I had taken prior in that things remained stable and unchanged. The good news was that there were no new lesions identified on this MRI and there were no adverse changes noted either. The less fortunate news was that there was no evidence that the Tysabri I had taken for the past twelve months had done anything to reduce or eliminate any of my existing lesions. And most notably, my overall condition remained relatively unchanged since I began my treatment with Tysabri in January 2011. "Well," I thought to myself, "it could be worse, the MRI results could have showed new lesions." So I accepted the results and decided to move forward.

After being off Tysabri for one month, Dr. Blitz and I spoke and explored new treatment alternatives for me. We made a decision that I would begin taking Copaxone daily injections of 20mg/ml. Simply putting it, Dr. Blitz explained to me that Copaxone worked by changing "bad guy" lymphocytes into "good guy" lymphocytes, and that these "good guys" (unlike with other MS therapies), crossed the blood-brain barrier into the central nervous system to suppress inflammatory activity. She also told me that unlike Avonex and other interferons used in the treatment of MS, Copaxone (which is not an interferon) did not have any adverse impacts on the liver or cause flu-like symptoms. Injection site reactions and flushing were generally the most common side-effects associated with the drug and were experienced by only a relatively small number of patients. "Wow," I thought to myself, "what a relief." I could actually take an MS drug without needing to worry about getting flu-like symptoms or experiencing spikes in my liver enzymes or run the risk of contracting PML!

Copaxone sounded novel to me and my enthusiasm peaked about beginning this new therapy, even though a daily injection was required in order to administer it. This was similar to how I felt whenever I started new MS therapies in the past—enthusiastic and excited. I was genuinely eager to begin Copaxone and remained hopeful that it would provide me with some noticeable symptom relief. While I didn't fully understand that "blood-brain barrier" thing, it sure sounded good and like the type of thing that might help make a difference. I silently imagined that my limp would improve, that my fatigue would dissipate, and that my balance would miraculously correct itself. And I would be able to say goodbye to my cane! I came back to reality when Dr. Blitz, as she did in the past whenever I began a new drug treatment, was very direct in saying that Copaxone (like other MS drugs that have been approved and were on the market at that time), was not a cure for MS or designed to eliminate symptoms and restore functionality. The drug was instead intended to halt or slow disease progression. Dr. Blitz clearly did her best to manage my expectations, as she had done in the past. "Each person is unique and as such may respond differently to different treatments," she would always tell me. That was enough to give me hope and keep me excited and optimistic that something good may happen.

I remained on Copaxone for nearly eighteen months and during this time I did not see any noticeable changes or improvements to my overall condition. If anything, my balance may have slightly worsened. Dr. Blitz attributed this more to the natural progression of the disease as opposed to the drug itself. In the time I was taking Copaxone, I had two MRIs done; one of the brain and one of the lumbar spine. Both of them, like the ones I had taken previously, showed the same thing:

> *There is stable appearance to the white matter plaques consistent with the patient's known history of Multiple Sclerosis. No new or enhancing lesions are seen. This examination is stable compared with the prior examination.*

During the time I was on Copaxone, I continued exercising regularly. I saw my personal trainer twice per week and went to the gym on my own another one/two times per week. I was probably in the best shape of my life since I had been exercising and training regularly for a few years now. I also continued with my six month "on again/off again" steroid treatments with Solu-Medrol, although now as time went on and with each set of infusions I received the lift that I got as compared to first time I started taking the steroids seemed to slowly lessen. Don't get me wrong, I still experienced a lift that lasted about four or five days but just not as great a lift as was compared to when I first started taking the steroids.

During the time I was taking Copaxone, going to the gym regularly and getting my steroid treatments, I also tried my hand at yoga. I attended yoga class religiously for a ninety minute session each Saturday morning. I continued with these Saturday morning sessions for about four months. Yoga was great in that it was very relaxing and offered me the opportunity to meet many nice people who also took the class. In fact, even my neurologist Dr. Blitz showed up at some of the yoga group sessions that I attended on Saturday mornings. While I was the only member of the group who had MS, for the most part I was able to keep pace with the class. I'm not sure I could say the same today. After giving yoga a try weekly for several months, I gave it up as I never really noticed that it had any real positive impact on my MS. Till this day though I occasionally use some of the breathing and relaxation techniques that I learned from my yoga classes to help me deal with stressful situations. Still though, I approached yoga with the same level of excitement and enthusiasm that I did each time I began a new drug or alternative treatment. And today I continue to search for that "silver bullet" that will ease and eliminate my MS symptoms. I remain confident and optimistic that someday I will find it!

After stopping yoga, I quickly started researching other complimentary alternative medicines, techniques, vitamins and supplements.

I dabbled for a few months in a crash diet of celery and horseradish (foods that different people had recommended), began taking probiotics by eating yogurt each morning and started taking a number of vitamin supplements. These included Vitamin D3, Magnesium, Calcium, Vitamin B-12 and Vitamin E. I also began taking Gingko Biloba twice per day in the hopes of getting a further energy boost. I then decided to try acupuncture. I was somewhat apprehensive and skeptical about this at first, as I was largely fearful of the pain that might be associated with being stuck with needles like a pincushion. I embarked on my acupuncture adventure with the same zeal and excitement that I did each time I started something new. I always wondered and thought to myself, "Would this be the silver bullet?" Surprisingly, acupuncture was not painful at all and my weekly forty-five minute therapy sessions were quite relaxing. I was fortunate in that the doctor recommended to me for acupuncture lived directly around the corner from my home in Jericho, Long Island, and practiced out of his home one day per week. In addition he had an office in New York City where he practiced a majority of the time. So, I did not need to make a special trip into the city each week to visit the doctor to get my acupuncture treatments. Therefore I had no excuse for not continuing with the weekly acupuncture regimen. Unlike some others I know who suffer from MS, I was not experiencing any pain so my experiment with acupuncture was solely aimed at improving my symptoms relating to gait and balance. Probably because it was so convenient and felt so relaxing, I stuck with acupuncture therapy for quite a few months even though my weekly visits were not covered by my medical insurance. In the spring of 2013, I stopped going for acupuncture treatment as I didn't see any real improvement in my overall condition. In addition, the expense started to add up and become more of a factor. Yes, it was very convenient and extremely relaxing; that must have had something to do with the low lighting and soft oriental music that played in my therapy room during each of my sessions. In large part though, because it wasn't really providing me with any noticeable benefit and was not covered under my medical insurance, I stopped going. Don't get me wrong. If I thought it was helping in the slightest, I would have continued with acupuncture treatments despite the fact that they were not covered by my medical insurance!

A few years later, I once again tried acupuncture – this time along with moxibustion (or "moxa" for short), a traditional Chinese medicine technique that involves the burning of mogwort, a small spongy herb used to facilitate healing. Based on a strong recommendation made by one of my NYC Express Bus commuting buddies, Janine, I gave this treatment a try. Specifically, Janine told me about her sister who had recently been diagnosed with Bell's Palsey (another neurological condition). Apparently after a few short acupuncture and moxa treatments with a highly recommended licensed carrier, her symptoms all but vanished. "Wow," I thought to myself, "this sounds great - I have nothing to lose by seeing this carrier and giving it a try." As of my writing of this manuscript, I continue with my acupuncture and moxa treatments. It is still too soon to see any results, and therefore I do not know yet if any benefits will eventually be realized. But, I remain hopeful!

My latest adventure has me drinking green juice each morning; I buy the pre-made bottled stuff, as it is much more convenient and easier than if I were to juice myself. While the bottled green juice does contain sugar, it is filled a number of all natural ingredients, including kale, spinach, celery, cucumber, etc. Since kale is often times referred to as "king of the garden," having a concoction that blends in a number of other greens rich in protein certainly cannot cause any harm (I think). I have also started drinking juice smoothies which are packed with a variety of nuts and fruits including things like almonds, blueberries, blackberries, raspberries, etc. The juice smoothies too contain sugar, but are also rich in protein and dietary fiber. While "yummy," these nutritional supplements are not cheap and average between five and seven dollars per quart. From a health perspective, I can only imagine these drinks are good for me. However, the jury is still out in terms of their having a positive impact on my MS.

In early 2013 I was driving in the neighborhood to pick up my dry cleaning and heard an interesting piece of information on the radio. An advertisement I guess, for Winthrop University Hospital that profiled a young woman diagnosed with MS several years prior who had to give up her passion for ballet dancing. The ad went on to mention that the young woman sought a fresh opinion and analysis of her disease, and began seeing Dr. Malcom Gottesman who was Director of MS treatment Programs at Winthrop University Hospital. The radio piece continued to profile the woman and said that after a few months of seeing Dr. Gottesman and pursuing a new treatment strategy, she began to feel better and started re-living her passion by resuming ballet dancing consistent with the routines she followed before being diagnosed with MS. The announcement on the radio piqued my interest momentarily, particularly since it mentioned Dr. Gottesman by name. He was one of the first doctors I saw in 2006 when I was trying to figure out what was wrong with me. The radio advertisement also highlighted the woman's stark improvement since she began visiting Dr. Gottesman at Winthrop. After the segment ended I basically forgot about it and continued going about my daily business. About a week later, I was driving to visit my dad at his house in Queens and heard the same segment again on the car radio. This time, I listened more attentively. But again, after the segment was over I virtually forgot about it. Later on that same day on the ride home from my dad's house I heard the segment *yet* again on the car radio. This time I thought to myself, "Wow, this is so weird. Could it be fate or is it just a strange coincidence?" I remember mentioning this to Luisa when I arrived home and her saying that it seemed interesting and that I should call Dr. Gottesman. "Call him," she said, "and make an appointment to see him. You have nothing to lose." We continued talking about it briefly for a few minutes and I remember telling Luisa I was perfectly satisfied with Dr. Blitz and really saw no reason to call Dr. Gottesman. She said she understood, but emphasized again that I had nothing to lose by calling him. She went on to say that maybe I should call because this could be some kind of omen since the same ad played on the radio three times within one week. I agreed with her that I had nothing to lose and that it was definitely strange that I heard the same radio advertisement several times in such a short period of time. So a few days later, I called Dr. Gottesman's office and made an appointment to go and see him later on that month when he had an opening.

In late February 2013 I went to see Dr. Gottesman. In the same building as he was in previously, he had moved into larger, much nicer office space on another floor. I guess business was good. I mentioned to Dr. Gottesman that the radio advertisement was the reason that prompted me to come see him for a second time. He chuckled, and I recall him saying in a low voice, "I guess the ad worked." He remembered me from my earlier visits in 2006 and told me that the radio piece I heard did represent an MS diagnosis for a person whose disease path was likely different than mine. He then went on to remind me that no two cases of MS for an individual is likely to be the same. Nonetheless, he said he would be happy to review my case and asked that I make a follow-up appointment to see him and bring with me at that time all prior MRI reports as well as my MS medical treatment history. He also gave me two scripts to have MRIs done of my brain and thoracic spine, with and without contrast, and said he would be happy to review with me the test results. He told me that he would also study my prior medical records to see if any changes to my current treatment regimen may be warranted. I thanked him and made it clear that I was simply interested in getting another [his] opinion and that I was quite comfortable with the care that I was receiving from my current neurologist, Dr. Karen Blitz. He said he clearly understood, knew Dr. Blitz well and told me that he was confident she was providing me with the best care necessary to treat my condition. Nonetheless he told me he would be happy to review my case and give me his opinion about my condition. As I left Dr. Gottesman's office, I stopped by the receptionist's desk and made a follow-up appointment to see him early the following month. In the meantime after I returned home, I scheduled the MRIs that the doctor ordered, gathered my past MRI reports and created a bullet point chronology of events summarizing my MS history which included a listing of the various medical treatments, vitamin supplements and alternative therapies that I had tried since being diagnosed with MS in July 2006.

Two weeks later in March 2013 I went to see Dr. Gottesman with copies of my prior test results in hand for him to review, along with a listing of the various treatments I underwent since my diagnosis and a chronology of my symptoms and notable events throughout my MS journey. The test results from the two MRIs ordered by Dr. Gottesman had been sent to him directly from the lab. Luisa came along with me to listen to what Dr. Gottesman had to say, and I'm sure to add things that I may have neglected to mention.

My follow-up appointment with Dr. Gottesman began with him again assuring me that he was certain that I was under the best care possible with Dr. Blitz, and that he understood my reasoning for seeking another opinion. He then gave me credit for proactively managing my disease, indicating that he wished more of his patients took such an active role in managing their disability. At that point I remembered why I thought so highly of Dr. Gottesman. He was a pleasant man, low keyed and down to earth and who spoke honestly, openly and sincerely. In terms of the most recent MRIs he prescribed I take, Dr. Gottesman told me that he received and reviewed the results, and they were indeed consistent with the results of past MRIs I had taken. Dr. Gottesman then listened as I took him through my MS history. He asked questions intermittently, took notes and occasionally looked at Luisa to gauge her facial expressions as I spoke (to be sure, I assumed, that I was accurately taking him through my medical history and event chronology and that I was not forgetting to mention anything critical). It appeared that I passed the test!

After spending nearly one hour with Dr. Gottesman, he said that it was his opinion that - as Dr. Blitz indicated - my MS was most likely now in the progressive phase. He went on to indicate that the evidence appeared to indicate that my MS may have been in the progressive phase since the onset of my diagnosis in 2006, since there were not a great number of relapses or pronounced exacerbations that occurred since that time. However, he emphasized that there was no way of being 100 percent certain about this since in fact there were some defined instances since being diagnosed where certain symptoms did become more pronounced, indicative of relapses that presumably then went into remission. He then stressed that I needed to remain mindful of the fact that none of the MRIs taken since my initial diagnosis, with one exception, showed any new or worsening lesion activities. In terms of my treatment, Dr. Gottesman went on to say that if I were his patient, he would be taking the exact same course of action that Dr. Blitz was taking and would not do anything differently at the current time. When Luisa and I then asked Dr. Gottesman what he suggested our next course of action be, he was very direct and told us, "While I would very much welcome you as my patient, I must tell you again that at this time I would not do anything different with your treatment than what Karen [Dr. Blitz] is currently doing, so therefore I'm not sure there is any valid reason for you to make a change." He went on to say that if he were in my shoes, he would continue with the current level of care, oversight and treatment being provided by Dr. Blitz. Before departing, I joked with Dr. Gottesman and said that I probably wouldn't be doing ballet dancing any time soon, referring to the woman profiled in the radio segment. As Dr. Gottesman smiled, I got up, shook his hand and thanked him for his time and told him that I would likely continue seeing Dr. Blitz. I did.

I continued with my daily Copaxone injections until the end of May 2013. Around that time I had a regularly scheduled quarterly appointment to see Dr. Blitz; here, she told me about a new oral drug called Tecfidera that had just recently received FDA approval. During my visit, I did not feel any need to mention to her that I went to see Dr. Gottesman for another opinion - so I did not. Dr. Blitz suggested that I try the drug Tecfidera, which was given in pill form and needed to be taken twice per day. Before I even asked (and she knew I would), Dr. Blitz told me that the most common side-effects of taking Tecfidera included feeling flushed and experiencing an occasional upset stomach; she indicated that no other side-effects associated with Tecfidera had been identified to date. She next told me that patients who took the medication with food were less likely to suffer from an upset stomach. She continued talking and told me that while taking the drug, she would order blood-work be done every four to six months to be sure my white blood cell count remained normal. Dr. Blitz then went on to say how studies that were done indicated that Tecfidera significantly cut relapses in half and reduced the risk of relapses by nearly fifty per-cent compared to placebo. From speaking with Dr. Blitz over the past year or so, it was becoming clearer to me that my condition was on the cusp of migrating from the relapsing remitting to the secondary progressive phase. The "relapses" I was now experiencing over the past couple of years were somewhat benign and relatively few. So I was curious why she was prescribing this new drug, Tecfidera, that was targeted to treat relapsing remitting MS.

Dr. Blitz told me that if anything I was probably correct in thinking that my MS was at the very beginning of the secondary progressive phase. She went on to tell me that Tecfidera had both anti-inflammatory and brain-protective characteristics, and that it did a number of different things to lower inflammation and lessen the ability of the immune cells to get in and attack the central nervous system. Additionally, she told me that Tecfidera showed evidence that it may also protect nerves from sustaining damage. Bottom line, she said, "everyone is different, the side-effects are minimal and therefore you have nothing to lose by trying it." This was similar to what she always told me in the past whenever she contemplated having me switch therapies. So true to form I remained excited and hopeful that this new therapy would have some noticeable impact on my symptoms, even though Dr. Blitz reminded me once again that Tecfidera, like other MS therapies that were on the market, was not necessarily designed to improve symptoms and restore functionality, but were rather intended to slow or halt disease progression. Prior to my starting to take Tecfidera, Dr. Blitz ordered a blood test to ensure that my white blood cell count was within normal range. The blood test results came back normal, and by July 2013 I had started taking the drug.

Over the next seventeen months or so I continued to take Tecfidera twice per day after meals, as prescribed. The convenience of taking the medication orally was great and sure beat the hassle of giving myself daily self-injections or even receiving monthly infusions. I know for some people however, the thought of giving oneself an injection prompted tremendous anxiety. For that reason alone I'm sure that the new oral MS medications (like Tecfidera) were deemed to be a godsend for many. For me however, the injection and infusion processes did not bother me. My reason for switching to this oral medication was purely related to my drive to try something new that might ultimately yield different and potentially more noticeable positive results. Some people subscribe to the mentality of "if it isn't broke, don't fix it." For me however, I will not rest until I have tried everything there is that can potentially help me overcome my disability.

During the time I was taking Tecfidera, my symptoms appeared relatively unchanged. Looking back from when I was initially diagnosed with MS, my gait did gradually worsen over the years and my fatigue also seemed to increase slightly, particularly toward the end of certain days. My balance became slightly more impaired too. Again, my neurologist Dr. Blitz told me that the progressive nature the disease was likely the cause. Meanwhile, each MRI I took annually showed that there were no new or enhancing lesions. Go figure. In the meantime, in the fall of 2013 I was beginning to develop some lower back pain. Both my primary care doctor and my neurologist told me this was more than likely related to the awkwardness of my gait and the fact that I was throwing my left foot out to the side each time I walked. Dr. Blitz prescribed the muscle relaxant Tizanidine for me. The drug offered me some temporary relief that was short lived. At one point, my back pain became so severe that I was unable to put pressure on my arms when using my walking cane. As such, one Sunday afternoon in November as I was getting out of my car returning from the grocery store and fell face down to the floor of my concrete driveway. I saw blood everywhere and was unable to get up or reach for my cell phone to call my wife for help. She was inside the house. At the top of my lungs I began screaming and yelling her name. "Help, Weezie (which is what I call her)... Weezie, help... WEEZIE! WEEZIE!!!"

I was scared. I was bleeding. I was cold. I could not get up. I knew I had hurt myself pretty badly, but I could not gauge the extent of my wounds. Thank goodness nothing was broken and I did not hit my head on the ground. I fell flat on my face instead and on my nose (thank goodness it was not broken). My lips and my chin took the brunt of the fall. I knew having a big nose would pay off someday, and it did. In all likelihood, my big nose helped break my fall! About a minute later (it was probably less than that, but seemed like it was a lot longer as I lay on the ground bleeding and screaming), Luisa came running out of the house. My neighbor Gary, who lives across the street, must have heard my screams from inside his house and also ran over. Luisa and Gary both helped me get up. I'm sure I was dead weight! They both grabbed me from under my arms and moved me inside my house. My face and nose were bruised and bleeding pretty badly, but I refused their offers to take me to the hospital for treatment since I didn't feel like I had broken anything. Besides, my cuts did not seem deep enough to warrant stitches. I eventually was able to convince Luisa and Gary that a trip to the hospital emergency room was not necessary. Back in 2013, urgent care walk-in centers essentially did not exist, so going to one was not an option. After Gary left, Luisa helped me clean up and bandaged my face. To put it mildly, I was quite shaken up and looked like a mess. My nose, chin and both my lips were swollen and bruised, my left cheek was badly scrapped and "black-and-blue" marks were starting to form under both of my eyes. I remained home that entire week and let nature take its course to heal my badly bruised face. Unfortunately, at the same time nature was taking its course on healing my battered face, it was also taking its course (in reverse) with my lower back. My lower back pain got progressively worse.

By the end of the week that Friday, the pain became so unbearable that I needed two cortisone shots to function. Luisa drove me to the doctor's office to get the shots. Within minutes after getting the injections, I felt immediate relief. While the pain relief was certainly very welcome, I knew that I eventually needed to do something to address the problem. I told my personal trainer Chris, whom I continued to see twice a week, about my back pain. He helped me slightly by developing a routine of stretching and weight exercises designed to ease my back pain and help me manage. I also began seeing a physical therapist that Chris recommended, but only for a short period of time. I was soon referred (by the physical therapist himself) to see the chiropractor (Dr. Brett Pastuch) who was co-located in the same office building that he was in. Initially, I began seeing Dr. Pastuch three times per week. After a few visits, my lower back pain became significantly better. The pain went from about a nine to a four (on a scale of one to ten), with ten being the worst. Within two months of seeing Dr. Pastuch, I was able to reduce my visits to once per week. To this day I continue to see Dr. Pastuch but now, twice per month. I have now made chiropractic visits part of my normal regimen. Thank goodness my back-pain has virtually disappeared, even with my altered gait. While I was not really a big believer in chiropractors before this, I can honestly say now that I would recommend chiropractic to anyone who may be experiencing severe back pain for which no other treatments have helped.

In November 2014, I went for one of my regularly scheduled visits with Dr. Blitz and told her I felt frustrated and wished there was something that could be done that would help improve my symptoms. The very slow but gradual progression of my symptoms was something I was determined to overcome. As I did each time I visited her, I would always half-jokingly ask Dr. Blitz the same question: "Have any cures been discovered yet?" This time though, I was more serious and Dr. Blitz sensed it. She asked me if I wanted to try another therapy and I told her I would try anything, within reason, that might help. She thought for a bit and then explained to me there was a drug called Rituximab (Rituxan for short), a form of chemotherapy that was approved for use in the treatment of certain lymphomas, leukemias, and other autoimmune disorders. She told me however, that it was still being tested for MS treatment and was not yet an approved MS therapy. She went on to explain to me that Rituxan was a monoclonal antibody that was given to some patients who had secondary progressive MS and that in one study, it showed improvement in patient symptoms and slowed further disease progression. I told Dr. Blitz that while this sounded great, the word "chemotherapy" scared me. "I like having hair," I told her. She laughed and said that for the dosage she would be prescribing for me (one initial infusion followed by another infusion nine to twelve months later), hair loss was not a side-effect that I needed to worry about. She went on to tell me that if anything, some of the more common side-effects may include things such as headache, fever, chills, nausea, rash or flushing. I trusted Dr. Blitz and figured that since in the past I agreed to try Tysabri (given the remote risk of contracting PML), agreeing to try Rituxan was a "no-brainer." I asked her quite bluntly what she would do if she was in my position, and without hesitation she said she would indeed try Rituxan. That was all I needed to hear, as I valued Dr. Blitz's opinion and had the utmost trust in her. So, I agreed to go ahead and try Rituxan. "One thing," she said, "since it is not an approved medication for treating MS, it may not be covered by your insurance." Nonetheless, she said her office would submit the approval request and would notify me of the results as soon as hearing of anything. In the meantime Dr. Blitz told me to stop taking my current medicine, Tecfidera, as I needed to be off it for at least thirty days before getting the Rituxan infusion.

A few weeks later Dr. Blitz's assistant Donna called to tell me that my insurance carrier denied the request for Rituxan, but that Dr. Blitz would be appealing the decision. Another three weeks went by and I received a letter from my medical insurance carrier indicating that my doctor's appeal was rejected and that they would not approve payment for the drug. "Not medically necessary" is what the letter said. The correspondence went on to indicate that there would be one final opportunity for me to personally appeal the decision. I was furious, and wasted no time in writing and sending a final appeal letter to my medical insurance carrier.

My appeal letter to the medical insurance carrier regarding their denial of Rituxan reads as follows:

The purpose of the letter is to formally appeal the Medical Director's decision to deny the infusion of Rituximab, 100 mg, on the grounds that it is not medically necessary for my condition.

For your reference, I have enclosed a copy of the denial letter issued on October 11, 2014. I was diagnosed with Multiple Sclerosis (MS) in the summer of 2006. Since that time, I have been under the treatment of Dr. Karen Blitz, and have been on various therapies, as summarized below:

> *Avonex: August 2006 - November 2008;*
> *Betaseron: January 2009 - December 2010;*
> *Tysabri: January 2011 - January 2012;*
> *Copaxone: February 2012 - June 2013; and*
> *Tecfidera: July 2013 - Present.*

During my last quarterly visit to Dr. Blitz in September 2014, I informed her that my balance and gait had worsened over the past 12 months. We determined that my disability, as measured by the EDS scale, had worsened form my previous score of 3 (moderate disability, with the ability to still walk), to a score of 5 (more severe disability, impairing my daily activities, and requiring assistance with walking). Today, I walk with the assistance of a cane. As a result, and in consideration of the various treatment methods I have been under since my 2006 diagnosis (as summarized above), Dr. Blitz prescribed Rituximab, explaining that it targets 'B' cells and is her suggested therapy for me in lieu of my current treatment (with Tecfidera). As MS is a very dynamic disease which affects everyone differently, I remain optimistic that Rituximab will have a positive impact on me. Dr. Blitz feels it is in my best interest to change my current treatment from

Tecfidera to Rituximab. I know she has already provided you with the appropriate documentation about my case to support her recommendation. In addition, my understanding is that total cost to the insurance company for Rituximab may be less than the costs associated with my current and prior treatments.

Given this cost factor, along with recommendation of my neurologist (Dr. Karen Blitz) who has been treating me since I was diagnosed 8 years ago, I am perplexed by the fact that the Medical Director at xxxxxxxxx (who has had zero interaction with me and is not at all familiar with my case) is denying this request for Rituximab.

While I am appealing this denial decision, I am also appealing to your sense of understanding and compassion. If the roles were reversed here and you were a victim of this horrible disease, wouldn't you follow the advice of your personal physician and welcome the use of a new form of therapy that just may improve your quality of life? I think we both know the answer!

I respectfully request that my appeal to this decision be reviewed, and that the denial decision be reversed. I look forward to hearing your decision shortly. In the interim, please feel free to contact either myself or Dr. Blitz should any further information be required.

Within four weeks of my sending this correspondence, I received a letter back from my medical insurance carrier that the decision to deny payment for Rituxan had been reversed. My letter worked! After the approval became final, I eagerly anticipated starting the drug. Administered via infusion, I remember being excited and optimistic as I headed to the infusion center, this time in Great Neck, Long Island, where I was told the treatment regimen would take approximately four to six hours. Like the time I received the Tysabri infusions, my infusion nurse (Regina) told me up front that there were going to be defined points throughout the process whereby the infusion drip would be temporarily stopped for a check of my pulse, blood pressure and other vital signs. About an hour after the Rituxan infusion started and Regina came back to check on me to take my vital signs, I told her I was becoming itchy and noticed an increasingly large rash spreading across my lower stomach. Almost immediately after telling her, Regina stopped the infusion. She quickly phoned Dr. Blitz who advised that the infusion should be completely halted. She was fearful that the allergic reaction I seemed to be having could impact my respiratory system and impede my ability to breathe freely. I was told that Dr. Blitz requested I remain at the infusion center for observation until my rash went away. I stayed at the center for a little over an hour until the itching stopped and the rash almost completely disappeared. Given my allergic reaction, I was certainly glad the infusion was stopped. The thought of my windpipe constricting and not being able to breathe freely scared me. At the same time though I was disappointed it was stopped, as I had high hopes Rituxan would have a positive impact on my symptoms. I guess the devil you know is a lot better than the devil you don't know!

The following week I went to see Dr. Blitz and discuss with her my next treatment option. Jointly we agreed that it probably made sense for me to go back on Copaxone, the treatment I was on a few years earlier that called for self-injection. However, in the eighteen months or so since I last took Copaxone, changes were made by the pharmaceutical company regarding the drug's dosage and administration. Instead of the need to inject the drug daily, the drug manufacturer came up with a 40mg/ml three times per week dosage. As the side-effects remained minimal and were basically unchanged since the last time I took Co-paxone, I had no hesitation proceeding.

Around the same time that I began taking Copaxone in January 2015, I learned from Dr. Blitz during one of my visits about a study done in Italy of men and women with mild-to-moderate MS symptoms who exercised at home with a Nintendo Wii-Fit balance board system. She told me about a twelve week study that was done on a group of people having MS which showed positive changes in areas of the brain responsible for balance and movement. The results of this study were compared to a group of people having MS who never used the Wii-Fit. "You should look into it," she said. My response to her: "Interesting. I'll check it out."

Later that day after I arrived home, I did some searching on the internet about what Dr. Blitz had told me. I found a piece that was published describing a study indicating researchers found that people having MS who did Wii-Fit balance training at home for thirty minutes per day, five days per week for thirteen weeks, had brain scans taken before and after doing balance training, with scans taken afterwards revealing an overall increase in brain plasticity. My continued "Googling" further showed that according to an article published in *Live Science* magazine by the study's Director Dr. Luca Prosperini, a neurologist at Sapienza University in Rome, Italy, [use of the Wii-Fit balance board] showed "improvements in myelin sheaths of nerves connecting areas of the brain involved in balance and movement, and [that these] improvements resulted in better nerve-signal transmission in these parts of the brain, resulting in the brain's ability to change its function or structure following training."

Wow. This sounded great! I did some further research and found that my neurologist, Dr. Blitz was actually quoted in an August 2014 edition of *Live Science* magazine saying: "I think this is a very important study for MS patients, because it showed scientifically that the brain can change in response to balance training." The article continued and contained a video clip that actually showed one of the physical therapists who initially treated me shortly after my diagnosis in 2006, Robert, talking about how he had been using the Wii-Fit balance board for about five years. He said it had helped him maintain and improve his balance, and that it provided him with real data showing his progress thereby keeping him motivated and interested in continuing to use it. One of the more revealing things which I learned from watching the video clip was something I never knew before. Robert, the physical therapist who treated me previously, actually had MS himself and that he had it when I was seeing him for treatment the 2006/2007 timeframe. I further learned from the piece that he was a patient of Dr. Blitz's.

No sooner did I finish reading the article and scrolling down the computer page did I look-up Robert's phone number, called and spoke to him. He actually remembered me as one of his past clients and gave me a full overview of his experiences using the Wii-Fit balance board. Robert could not say enough positive things about the system. He answered all my questions and wholeheartedly recommended I get and start using it. Double wow! I was sold!! So what did I do? I purchased it. I spoke with Luisa and the next day we made an online purchase from eBay of the Wii-Fit system with the balance board. Two days later it arrived to my home via Federal Express.

For the first month after it was delivered, admittedly it sat unused in the box in which it was shipped. Other than Luisa hooking up the system and testing it to be sure it worked, I really didn't start using it right away. This was despite the fact that Luisa "nagged" me repeatedly throughout the month to begin spending time using it. Several weeks later (I guess the "nagging" worked), I began using the system four or five times per week and played a variety of different balance "games." Not only was it fun, but it was somewhat addictive. I liked the fact that it showed the score of my current session and compared it with the scores I achieved in my previous ten sessions. That just made me even more "competitive" with myself and further motivated me to improve and beat my last score. And because the system had the same balance "games" in both a "beginner" and "advanced" mode, I was able to toggle back and forth between the two difficulty levels and further challenge myself. I sometimes use the Wii-Fit system today, although not as consistently as when I first got it. I use it as an adjunct to being active (i.e. going into NYC for a majority of the workweek, continuing my weekly exercise routines at the gym, seeing my personal trainer, etc.). And just like in the past whenever I tried anything new and different, I remain optimistic that the Wii-Fit balance board would provide me with a great benefit. I am excited and hopeful that using the Wii-Fit will over time help me improve my balance. I silently imagine that I will eventually become steadier when walking and on my own two feet. Has it made any difference to date? Nothing noticeable – only time will tell. Admittedly though, I slacked-off from using it about six months after starting – I need to get back "with the program."

Around the same time that I stopped taking Tecfidera, switched to Copaxone and started using the Wii-Fit, I began my six month "on again/off again" steroid treatment. It was also time for me have my annual MRI taken. When I went for the MRI this time I noticed that it took about half the time as it did in the past—about twenty minutes compared to forty to fifty minutes it took previously. As I was leaving the imaging facility I commented to the clinician about the shortened duration of the test and was informed that new and more powerful machinery was recently installed that offered more advanced imaging technology, thereby shortening the duration of the testing and also allowing for more detailed and robust images. I smiled and thought to myself that scientists and researchers were making advancements all around when dealing with MS. Not only were they coming-up with new medications and treatment options at a rapid pace, but they were also enhancing imaging techniques to further improve diagnostic capabilities.

As in the past, the MRI done this year once again showed that there was no change from the exam I took twelve months earlier.

> *Compared the MRI taken in January 2014, there is stable imaging of findings of demyelinating disease. No MRI signs of active demyelination. No new white matter lesions.*

I guess I need to be thankful that things continued to remain stable and that there are no new lesions or signs of active demyelination. My goal now is to remain stable and be in top condition until the cure is found. Despite this, I continue to try new and different treatment therapies and techniques in the hopes of finding that "silver-bullet."

Something I have not yet looked into but plan to research further is equine therapy, or therapeutic horseback riding. I heard about this and have actually read a few articles about how equine therapy has been shown to provide people with impaired mobility caused by MS and other neurological conditions increased balance, improved muscle control and enhanced strength. One study which I read talks about how horseback riding gently and rhythmically moves the body in a manner similar to a walking, and that people with MS undergoing equine therapy have been shown to benefit from it. Specifically, MS patients developed increased confidence, became more independent and had greater self-esteem. I know that Ann Romney, wife of 2012 presidential candidate Mitt Romney who suffers with MS, has indicated on several occasions that horseback riding helped her "gain back her core strength and balance."

So like I have always done, I will look further into this complimentary alternative therapy, equine therapy, to see if in fact it is something beneficial for me to try. I'm sure that in addition to equine therapy, other complimentary alternative medicines and therapy techniques will continue to surface that I will look into and try in an effort to help improve my gait, balance and strength. It should be fairly obvious to all those reading by now that I will continue being relentless in my pursuit of potential medicines and therapies that may improve my MS symptoms. That is of course assuming there are no significant adverse side-effects!

Chapter 12

Limitations…What Limitations?

S ince being diagnosed with MS in 2006, I have begun realizing that there were many things in life that I could no longer do like I once did. Granted it took me a few years to realize this, but as time has gone by I've become more of a realist. Don't get me wrong, there are still times when I feel like I can do anything or go anywhere. It must have a little to do with wanting to feel "macho," something I'm sure all guys experience. But there is no longer a day that goes by that I haven't resigned myself to the fact things are different now. There are many bigger things in life that I simply can no longer do. Things like not being able to play sports (not that I was ever that good at sports and played that frequently anyway), go bicycle riding, walk along a sandy beach, occasionally go out for a jog, undertake large projects (like cleaning the attic, or cleaning out the garage, or painting, etc.), wash and wax the car, putter around in the garden, go grocery shopping, walk about in a mall, etc. These are some of the things that I have recently grown reluctantly accustomed to *not* being able to do. While it has taken me a while, for the most part I have come to grips with this reality. As is often said, "It is what it is."

However, it is many of life's everyday things that are normally taken for granted that I have difficulties with. It is hard for me to do them, and that bothers me a great deal! Not being able to do the seemingly simple things, or taking longer to do them, continues to frustrate me on a daily basis. Some days I become so frustrated that I let out a big scream, and yes still occasionally yell out, "Why me?" Often times I loudly shout-out some weighty profanities (when I am alone, of course). After I take a deep breath, dust myself off and face head on the reality of the situations at hand; I say to myself, Why _not_ me? and start thinking of ways to devise simple workarounds (most of the time) to help lessen my constraints and limitations. When I finally figure out a "workaround" and am able to at least partially do the task I set out to do, I feel a sense accomplishment. But there are some tasks for which there are no workarounds that I am just unable to perform (at least for the time being), or have more difficulties doing. On days when this happens, a dramatic scream or shout-out is usually _not_ the norm. What is the norm are the low mumbling curses I cobble together and say under my breath. I try not to show it, but I can never forget that having MS does suck! However, I do my best to take one day at a time and move forward. The loss of independence, diminished self-confidence and weakened self-esteem are feelings that I have every day. This sucks! One thing is for certain though, I will not give up and let this horrible disease called MS win!

I constantly try to figure out ways to make life easier for myself when undertaking daily activities. I think about not dwelling on the difficulties associated with doing certain things and I figure it may be worthwhile for some people to hear me talk about them, the workarounds or steps I have taken and other stuff I have done to make life easier and help me cope. Hence, this is the reason behind and the purpose for me writing this chapter. Here are a few examples:

Setting the clock on my nightstand one hour ahead. This may
sound trivial and archaic, but it works! While I set my alarm clock
for the "normal" hour, it actually goes off one hour earlier than the
real time due to my setting the time ahead. After a while this has
become easy for me to get used to, and my body clock has now become accustomed to it. Granted, it absolutely drives Luisa crazy.
Whenever we are in the bedroom, she will often ask me what the
real time is. But for me, doing this very simple act psychologically
helps me ensure that I remain on-time, avoid rushing and never
run late. I quickly forget that I have moved the clock ahead and
have an extra hour of time, particularly when I hurriedly glance
over at the clock on my nightstand each morning. At the start of
each day this gives me the extra time I need to shower, dress and
eat breakfast. It also allows me to get ready without hurrying and
stressing out. As simplistic as this may sound, it helps a great deal
and I recommend trying it!

Laying out my clothes the night before. A few years after I was diagnosed with MS and began exhibiting symptoms, I noticed that it
was becoming more of a challenge each morning searching my
dresser in the dark for socks, underwear and clothes to wear without
tripping or turning on the lights and awakening Luisa. As time went
on and after a few stumbles, I began to realize that there had to be
a better way. So I began getting my clothes and other accessories
together after dinner the night before and laying them out on my
nightstand. It has become so much easier doing this before going
to bed with the lights on versus doing it in the morning when it's
still dark. It has also eliminated for me some of the stress associated
with contemplating at the last minute what to wear as I get ready
each morning. Whether laying-out my work clothes, my gym attire
or my street clothes I have made the "night before layout" part of

my normal regimen for a few years now. As this too may sound like something simplistic and trivial, it really does help!

<u>Running those Saturday morning errands.</u> Running errands is something that I still try to do whenever I can. I am usually reluctant to ask Luisa or my daughters for help. This is not because I am afraid they will say no, but in large part it is due to the fact that I do not wish to bother them. Besides, doing the "little things" helps me feel more useful, gives me a greater sense of independence and makes me feel like I am less of a burden to others. I guess I'm just a stubborn Italian and am too proud to ask for help! Most times, if Luisa sees me getting ready to go out, she will ask where I'm going. When I tell her she says things like "leave everything, I'll drop off and pick up your clothes at the cleaners later," or "leave the checks on the counter and I will go to the bank in a little while to cash them," etc. Granted, there are some days when I just don't have the "oomph" to get up and leave the house. On these days I generally take her up on the offer or will occasionally ask for a favor whenever I'm not approached for help. It took me a while to ask for help, but nearly ten years after being diagnosed with MS my "shyness" has virtually disappeared. When I do leave the house to run errands, I have started opening my eyes and have begun noticing and taking advantage of some things that are available to make life easier. For example, I found a dry cleaner that offers drive-up service. It *does* cost about twenty-five cents more to dry-clean each garment, but the extra cost is well worth it as not having to get out of the car is a huge help to me. Another example is going to the bank. I would always park the car in the Citibank parking lot and walk inside the branch or the vestibule housing the ATM machine to do my banking business. A few years ago I noticed there was a Citibank branch located nearby my house with a drive-up window. This is some-

thing that was always there, but it is something that I never before paid any attention to. Not having to get out of the car to do my banking business was something I normally took for granted in years past. Today however, this has suddenly become very important and helpful to me now that I have MS. Needless to say I now always use the drive-up window. Again, this may seem like a small thing but to me it is huge. I no longer need to ask a family member for a favor and say something like "Hey, would you mind stopping at the bank for me?" Now, I can do it myself! If I could offer advice to anyone reading this who has MS, instead of saying, "I can't do that" (unless you really physically cannot) think a little more creatively and outside the box to see if there are things that you can avail yourself to which may possibly make it easier to run errands and do those daily chores. At a minimum this helps to remove any excuses for not "getting out there" and staying active. Also, this does wonders for my self-esteem!

Pumping gas. In the past I never hesitated to pull up to the pump, get out of my car, walk inside to see the gas station attendant, hand him money and say, "$25 of regular on pump 6." I'd then walk outside to my car and pump away. This very simple task became more of a chore as my MS symptoms slowly progressed. Getting out of the car, walking inside to pay the gas station attendant and then walking back to my car to "pump away" had become a big challenge for me. Today I still pump my own gasoline but instead of walking forty + yards to see and pay an attendant and then walk back to my car, I take full advantage of the debit card payment mechanism located right on the pump. I guess the walk I did in the past was good for me, even though I could have taken advantage of the debit card device on the pumps that did exist back then. Besides, in my "younger days" I perceived it to be a sign of laziness by not getting out of the car and walking inside to pay the attendant. Plus it was a good opportunity for me to pick up a candy bar, a bag of chips or a soda! Today though the ability to pay at the pump is a blessing in disguise, as it allows me to exercise just another small bit of independence by not having to rely on others to do a relatively simple daily task like going to the gas station and fueling my car. Besides, the candy bars, chips and sodas were all things I could certainly do without!

<u>Helping with the dishes</u>. I always felt somewhat guilty by the fact that Luisa would normally prepare a nice dinner each evening. Yes, she certainly is a great cook! I would eat up a storm each evening and then when we were all done, I'd watch her at the sink cleaning the dishes or load them into the dishwasher. Not being very domesticated, I figured the least I could do was to help with the dishes. A few years after being diagnosed with MS and as my symptoms began to worsen, there were certain days that standing up in front of the sink to do the dishes was certainly a challenge. And there were also days when I felt like I had no energy at all to help cleanup. Luisa would always say things like, "Just leave everything in the sink and I'll clean the dishes later or tomorrow morning," or "The dishwasher is dirty so leave everything and I will load it and clean up later." For a while I complied with her wishes. Lately however, I have come to realize that by simply moving one of the kitchen-island stools over to the front of the sink, I am able to sit and more easily do the dishes. This presents less of a challenge for me since I can now sit down when I do them as opposed to standing up. I also feel a lot better being able to say things to Luisa like, "Go sit down, relax and watch television. I'll clean up and take care of the dishes." Plus believe it or not, doing the dishes and cleaning-up the kitchen makes me feel good and more useful.

<u>Doing my "Target run" and going to the supermarket</u>. Another thing that makes me feel useful is keeping busy by going out and fetching things at the store. Almost every time that I venture out to a store, Lusia tells me to "stay home" or asks, "What do you need? I'll go." She clearly means well and is being sympathetic to some of the mobility limitations and balance issues that I have which are the result of my having MS. Her benevolent offers to help should not get me upset, but they sometimes still do! Many times I snap back. I don't mean to snap, but I _do_ and say in a short, angry and abrupt manner, "No, I'll go." I'm sure this upsets her, as she frequently will walk away and let out a big sigh. At times it's almost as if her offers to help make me feel like an invalid of sorts. I resent feeling like I am inept! But after a few seconds I realize this is not her intention. She is _not_ saying these things to make me feel inept or incompetent. On the contrary, she is trying to help and support me. However, at _that_ moment it's too late, as I have already snapped back. As time has gone on though, I have become more understanding and have tried to take the edge off my response. Now I will usually respond with things like, "That's okay, I feel like going," or "Thanks for offering, but I'd rather go and will probably call you on the phone when I return home and pull the car into the driveway so you can come outside of the house and help [me] carry in the bags." There are times when I'm not really feeling that strong and full of energy, so I take her up on her offer and say things like, "Okay, thanks, that's great. As long as you don't mind going to the store for me." Granted, on occasion I may still snap back. But, I am a lot more conscious of my responses now and try very hard to temper my tone. God knows I try! And sometimes when no one is at home, I'll just decide on a whim to take a ride and do one of my infamous "Target runs."

Believe it or not, something as simple as going to the store is quite therapeutic for me. Thanks to my dad's suggestion a few years after I was diagnosed with MS, I applied for and got a handicap placard for my car. So now I can go outside to a store and park my car in the handicap parking spaces which are always in front of the entrance to most stores. Once I park the car, I head straight for a shopping cart which really serves as a "walker" for me so that I can go up and down each aisle at my leisure. One of my favorite stores to frequent is a nearby Target that carries about everything imaginable. Whenever I go there I usually wind up filling up a shopping cart, often times with things that we either do not immediately need or unbeknownst to me with things that Luisa has already purchased in one of her recent trips to the market. Paper towels and toilet paper seem to always top my list, and I generally "stock up" on these items. After I make my way to the checkout and I pay for the merchandise, which is then bagged and placed back in the shopping cart for me (I always request the check-out person to pack things lightly and use multiple bags), I walk outside to the car and slowly remove the bags from the cart and place them in the trunk or in the back seat. This activity presents the biggest challenge for me. It takes me a lot of time. Sometimes another patron walking to their car will offer to assist me. Of late, rather than dismiss and turn-down their offers for assistance, I have begun to proudly accept them. When I return home, I keep my promise and call Luisa from outside in the driveway on my cell phone and request she come outside and help me bring the bags inside the house. I have no choice, since carrying bags and simultaneously juggling for balance with my cane is usually not very easy. When we are done bringing the bags inside the house and placing the contents onto the kitchen island, many times Luisa will say things like, "Why did you buy this?" or "We have paper dishes, you didn't need to buy them and besides I have no room in the cupboard to put them," or "Do you think we have enough yogurt?" I have since learned to just smile and not say anything that may prompt an argument. Before calling on my cell phone and asking Luisa to come out of the house and help, I oftentimes "smuggle" a big package of toilet paper or paper towels from my car into the garage. These items are light so I'm still able to remove them from the car and transport them relatively easily. After all, these are amongst my "favorite" items to purchase!

On occasion I'd return home from the store when no one was home. That's because when I left the house earlier in the day I decided on a whim to do my "Target run" without telling anyone I was going, since there was no one home at the time to tell without verifying anyone would be there when I returned. Hence when I would return home there was no one to call from the driveway to ask for help with carrying the bags inside. I've learned the hard way that leaving the house and going to stores on a whim with no one at home is _not_ something advisable for me to do. Therefore, this is something that I've only done once or twice. Unloading the bags from the car and carrying them inside the house is a very lengthy and taxing task for me, so this is not something I generally make a habit of doing any more. "So what's the big deal," one might ask? My answer is simple: It is truly a struggle for me to carry the bags inside the house from the car, carry them up the stairs of our high ranch house and place them on the kitchen island. Plus there are always lots of bags to carry due to the request I'd make to the checkout cashier to "pack lightly" and use extra bags; therefore there are a lot more trips to make back-and-forth between the house and the car. Without exaggeration, it probably takes me alone just as much time bringing the bags inside the house from the car as it does versus the amount of time I spend at the store shopping. So I now very rarely leave the house to do my "Target runs" unless I confirm that someone is planning to be home when I return.

Yes, going out to the store makes me feel good and it serves as my "therapy" session for the day. Thank goodness for shopping carts though, as they always help me navigate up and down the store aisles. A few times though I had to go back to the store to retrieve my cane that I inadvertently left in a shopping cart. I cannot wait for the day when forgetting my cane in a shopping cart becomes a conscious decision and does not create a need for me to go back to the store and retrieve it.

<u>Buying cold-cuts and redeeming recyclables:</u> On some Sunday afternoons I will also make my way to the local Shop-Rite supermarket to buy cold cuts and other goodies to pack for lunch for the upcoming work-week. In addition, every other month or so I will take a few plastic garbage bags from my garage that are filled with empty bottles and cans and drive over to the local Waldbaum's for insertion of them one by one into the recycling machines for the .5 cent deposit. But instead of carrying the plastic bags filled with the recyclables by hand inside to the store's "Bottle & Can Redemption Center," I make it easy for myself by dumping the bags filled with recyclables from the trunk of my car into a shopping cart; I then proceed inside. Again, thank goodness for shopping carts! Retrieving the recyclables for the five-cent deposit isn't the point, but getting out of the house and doing something is!

So by using something as simple as a shopping cart to hold onto, I have figured out a way to get out to stores and walk around. There are some days that I don't really need to buy anything. Hence there is no real need for me to go the store, let alone the need to wheel around a shopping cart once I get there. However as I've said before, getting out and going to the store is my "therapy" and grabbing a shopping cart (or my "walker") makes strolling throughout the store or the supermarket much easier. Plus, wheeling around a shopping cart is seemingly very inconspicuous. It allows me to walk around and "fit right in" without wielding a walker and having a flashing neon red light attached to my back saying, "I am disabled."

The chore of showering daily. There are some daily grooming tasks like showering, shaving, drying my hair, etc., where a number of simple techniques and devices can be used to make things a little easier. Basic things like installing a grab-bar in the shower, putting a small stool or bench there in the shower to sit on, placing a non-slip matt on the floor or installing a handheld shower message are all important safety items that can also be very helpful. For me, having a grab-bar is about all I currently need and rely on. But I also have a small stool placed in the shower just in case I lose my balance and need to sit. Thank goodness that to date this is not something that has occurred all that often. My goal is to get into and out of the shower as quickly as possible each morning. I'd say that on average it takes me about ten minutes to disrobe, get into and out of the shower and dry off. That's probably about six or seven minutes longer than it took in my Pre-MS days. This added time relates to the conscious effort I make to turn and move more slowly and deliberatively in order to avoid slipping and falling. The extra few minutes it takes me to get into and out of the shower each morning may not sound like a lot, but it makes a big difference for me when getting ready for work in the mornings. This is one of the reasons I set my clock ahead to ensure I have extra "get-ready" time and do not need to rush. To date, I am fortunate in that I have not had any slips or falls when showering. And it is only on very rare occasions when I'm having a bad balance day that I need to sit on the stool to complete my shower. Afterwards, I step out of the shower to dry off, shave, brush my teeth and dry my hair. As I do this I lean the lower torso of my body lightly on the sink so that I do not lose my balance while standing in front of the bathroom mirror. During this time that I remain standing, I am determined not to give in and make things easier for myself by sitting. While on some days it is tempting for me to sit at times, I do not. I consider my morning routine a prerequisite or a warm-up to "rev my engine," keep me moving and get me set to go out and about each day. Between showering, shaving, brushing my teeth, drying my hair and getting dressed it takes me on average about fifty minutes to "get ready." That's about twice as long as it would probably take for a person without MS to get ready.

Placing the garbage pails out by the curb. Early each Monday and Thursday morning trash collection in Jericho occurs. On Fridays, the recyclables are also collected. So that means that on the nights before, the trash cans and the recycle bin which sit on the side of the house need to be dragged down the driveway and placed out by the curb. The majority of the time I'm basically the only one in the house that remembers. As such, I draw the short straw and have the arduous task of putting out the garbage pails. On rare occasions, I am pleasantly surprised when I pull up into the driveway and see the pails have already been put out by the curb—compliments of Luisa. Most times though, I am the lucky one that remembers. Placing the garbage pails and the recycle bin out by the curb are not always "top-of-mind" items which Luisa generally thinks of doing. But me, being the anal retentive one, I never forget. Prior to my having MS, placing the pails out by the curb the night before garbage pickup was a simple task that I generally did without giving a second thought to. As my MS progressed and my balance worsened, dragging the pails to the curb was something that I really dreaded doing. A few years back when the garbage pails were worn and it was time to replace them, Luisa and I smartly purchased pails with wheels on the bottom so dragging them (now rolling them) from the side of the house to the curb was much easier for me. We purchased new pails with wheels on them rather unknowingly and never factored my having MS into the purchase decision. Nonetheless, that simple "workaround" continues to be a tremendous help to me. This is just another example of how such a simple thing allows me to continue doing an everyday task that helps me to remain feeling useful.

Sitting out by the pool and taking in some sun. After I was diagnosed with MS in the summer of 2006, I remember on summer weekends sitting in a lounge chair taking in the sun out by the pool in my house in East Hampton. After an hour or so of lounging in the hot sun, I remember getting up and making my way over to the pool to take dip; I often felt wobbly (almost as if I were drunk). There were also times I recall climbing up onto a rubber float in the pool to lay out and sunbathe. After about thirty minutes or so of lying on a latex rubber float in the hot sun, it was time to get out of the pool, make my way inside to my air-conditioned house for a reprieve from the heat and get a drink of cold water. As I was walking and went inside, I again had the same wobbly and drunkard feeling. I quickly learned that the sun and the heat were not friends to MS. This was something which I heard previously but did not (or did not want) to believe. It was something that I was unwilling to accept. But I soon figured out that something I always did, sunbathing, would become a thing of the past. Great. I couldn't sit out in the sun by the pool nor could I sunbathe at the beach, since walking and standing in sand is _not_ something that my MS allows me to do. My intolerance to heat was real. Feeling wobbly and unbalanced, as if I were drunk, was not fun. Interesting though...when I was younger and back in college I remember paying to feel that way! So much for enjoying summer time in the Hamptons during the new millennium!

The following year I discovered and purchased a float that had a rubber tube around the perimeter that boarded and supported a mesh bottom. I was able to take in the sun by lying in the float and because of the mesh bottom, my body was partially submerged in the cool water. Once "on board," I was able to lay back and relax, listen to a classic rock playlist on my iPod and soak-in the sun. Also I would frequently dangle my feet and legs from the float into the water in order to get-in some very basic aquatic exercise. This was great! I was able to get my daily dose of Vitamin D by sunbathing, hang out and relax in the pool, listen to my favorite tunes on my iPod and exercise! Because the cool water "rejuvenated" my body, I felt normal when getting off the float and out of the pool to walk around. Not only did I *not* feel wobbly and off balance, I actually felt refreshed and could swear that for an hour or so afterwards I was able to move around and walk faster with greater balance and stability. Luisa would usually make a comment about this as well. Now I was able to drink a beer or two or have a glass of wine and experience feeling wobbly and "drunk" on purpose! And sometimes for short periods after getting out of the pool, I was able to walk without the cane. Wow!

To this day I use my mesh float each summer to enjoy the pool and take in the sun's rays. Of course my SPF 30 sunblock is always nearby. Call it a "workaround" but I have found a way to enjoy something I thought my MS had taken away—relaxing in the pool on a hot summer sunny day. Plus, the Vitamin D that comes from the sun is often written about as being a positive supplement recommended for people having MS. This is a medicinal "win-win"! Who would have known that my mesh float would have therapeutic value!

In addition to some of the tasks I talk about above where I was able develop workarounds and improvise in order to make things a little easier, as I've pointed out there are some tasks that I simply cannot do or where improvisation is not an option. There are also tasks that are tempting which I sometimes try to do as well as everyday tasks that I have no choice doing that present big challenges for me. Granted it *does* take me longer to do these things versus the time it would take an average person without MS to do them. But I continue to persevere and constantly tell myself that "if it takes me a little longer" or "if I cannot do it," so be it.

Here are a few examples:

<u>Shoveling snow and walking in the snow and ice</u>. I hate when it snows and I have to watch helplessly from inside the front window of my house as Luisa navigates the snow blower/snow shovel down the sidewalk, across the driveway and over the front stairs. I watch as she removes the snow from our car. I feel feeble and sad as I gaze out the window. More often than not I feel like "less of a man." This is probably one of the most frustrating things I have to deal with. Talk about taking a blow to my self-esteem!

Speaking of the snow, I find myself powerless being stuck inside the house whenever it snows and sleets. The sidewalks and streets that are covered with ice and snow make it very dangerous for me to go outside on many winter days, and sometimes prevent me from going into the city for my business. With my balance being off, slipping and falling is not that difficult for me to do. And I don't need any help from "Mother Nature" to do it! When the temperatures warm up on some winter days and the snow and ice begins to melt, I will venture into the city. However, I exercise extreme caution as to where I step and also where I lean and press my cane on the ground to avoid icy pavements and terrains. A few

Christmases ago, Santa bought me a pair of slip-on rubber shoe grips with cleats. I call these my "snow tires," and they actually do make a difference when I walk outside. They prevent me from slipping and falling on the snow and ice. Without them I would be totally "shut in" on very wintery days. However, this relatively inexpensive ($9.99) accessory or "workaround" allows me to at least venture outside and go to work on most winter days.

Exercising at the gym. Going to the gym also continues to present a challenge for me. Granted it is easier for me to stay inside and not venture outside for a workout on cold winter days. However, I am determined to not forgo my exercise routines and will do whatever it takes to make it to the gym. As time went on and my MS slowly progressed, I found it increasingly more difficult to walk from my car and into the elevator to get inside the fitness center. The facility does have formal designated handicapped parking spots in front of the building (although this is "makeshift" handicapped parking, with a few handicapped placards placed in the front of only three regularly sized parking spaces that are adjacent to the front of the building). I'm not sure how people who use wheelchairs are expected to get into and out of their cars. To add to the challenge, there are several stairs which lead from the parking lot to the building's entrance. And up until 2014, there was no ramp. I'm not particularly good at going down stairs and after a while I began to get pissed off each time I would leave the gym. For me, going up stairs presents *less* of a challenge than does going down stairs—particularly after working out. A year or so later toward the end of 2014 I called the President and CEO of the sport club facility a few times to voice my concerns. My calls went unanswered and the messages I left were not returned. A few weeks later I put my concerns in writing and sent them in an email to the club's President and CEO. Another two weeks went by, and I did not get any response to my email. So I called again and this time left a left a pretty strong and direct voice message. I also sent another email, this one more potently worded than the one which I sent previously. In a nutshell I indicated that I was disappointed that there was no response to any of my prior communications, and that the company had until the end of the following week to have someone contact me before I registered a complaint with the U.S. Department of Justice responsible for administering the Americans with Disabilities Act (ADA). I did this out of frustration, and it was less of an ultimatum but more of an attempt to spur the company to action. A few days later I got a response directly from the office of the NYSC President and CEO. What a surprise! Less than one month after that, a handicapped ramp began being constructed and installed leading from the parking lot into the facility of the sports club. Within a few weeks, the ramp was complete. Leaving the gym now became much easier for me and I assume for other disabled patrons as well. I guess it's true that "the squeaky wheel gets the grease"—hear that, Dad? I know that my father would be proud of me!

My workouts at the gym now take about ninety minutes to complete. A few years ago, they took about sixty minutes to complete. For the most part this is due to the extra time it takes me to walk inside the gym from one piece of equipment to another. You see, the facility is spread out and quite large. There is no workaround for this! I'm not complaining though, as the facility is clean, big, uncluttered, laid out very well and has a wide variety of fairly "new" equipment. I also quite often take a short rest before moving from one piece of exercise equipment to another, so this adds further to the total amount of elapsed time that I spend at the gym. The good news is that what used to be a challenge for me when leaving the gym due to the absence of a handicapped ramp leading from the building to the parking lot is now no longer an issue.

233

<u>Getting my hair cut</u>. About once a month I drive over to a salon near my house to get my hair cut. I have been seeing the same haircutter, Ralph for about a dozen years now. Ralph has always been very good about giving me the assistance I need when navigating from the shampoo area to his barber chair, which is on the complete opposite side of the salon. I remember telling Ralph a few years after I was diagnosed that I had MS. This was probably the first time I walked into the salon with a cane. I remember Ralph's reaction being somewhat muted. He told me that he surmised something was wrong since he had seen me limping for quite some time and that after a few months he started doubting my story that I had hurt my knee. He also told me that someone he knew who went to the same gym as I recognized me, often saw me struggling and said something to him. At this point, I had to be honest with Ralph and "come clean." I must say though that from the time I disclosed my condition to him, Ralph was and continues to be great and always does his best to assist me—but only when he feels I need it. He does not go "over the top" and never treats me like an invalid. I appreciate this immensely!

The hair salon is about a five minute five drive from my house and I am always able to park in either a handicap space or in a parking spot in the lot directly across and pretty close to where the salon is located in a small strip mall. Plain and simple, there is no "workaround" or creative way to make getting a haircut easier; unless of course I cut it myself—something that I am not about to do! Funny because I probably could have arranged a while ago for Ralph to come to my house once a month to cut my hair. I have never asked him to do this though and unless I am absolutely unable to leave the house, I never plan to. Leaving the house to get my hair cut is just another small thing that keeps me moving and makes me feel good. I know, this must sound somewhat odd. But it's true!

<u>Getting up and walking over to my colleagues in the office to talk</u>. There is really no "workaround" for walking over and having a discussion with my work colleagues to talk or ask a question, unless I chose to scream out and disturb everyone else working in the office. This is *not* a practice I generally do. Whenever I had a need to speak urgently with one of my colleagues or business my partners, I would get up and make my way over to their cubicles which were located about thirty yards from me on the far side of the office. (Ultimately, we moved into new office space and made certain that our cubicles were positioned adjacent to and within earshot of one another). Prior to this, for non-urgent matters I would email, telephone or text them asking that they please come over to me when they had a chance. I often thought of moving my workspace closer to them at the far side of the office, but never chose to do this since my current location was just a few hundred feet from the elevator entrance, the restroom, the water cooler and nearby to the photocopier. It was also a few hundred feet from the conference rooms which we used for teleconferencing and to hold client meetings. I guess one could say I was sitting in the "high-rent" district, the "Park Avenue" of office space. There was just too much to give up and trade-off in a move so I continued to remain where I was. Plus, I always had a special fondness for Park Avenue!

<u>Commuting into Manhattan via the Express Bus versus using the Long Island Rail Road</u>. As I discuss in an earlier chapter, I was indeed fortunate to have discovered in 2011 an Express Bus service that allowed me to stop commuting into Manhattan via the Long Island Rail Road. Climbing up and down the stairs to the LIRR train platform had become difficult for me. The elevators frequently did not work and when they did, they often smelled like a soiled rest room at the Bronx Zoo. So initially taking the Express

Bus made it much easier and much more humane for me to commute from Long Island into New York City. The commuter bus service offers free Wi-Fi service and operates full size "luxury" coach buses. The company runs separate downtown and midtown routes, with the downtown bus making its last stop just two blocks away from the American Express building at the World Financial Center where I was consulting at one time. As far as commuting goes, taking the Express Bus versus taking the LIRR is "hands-down" better. There is no comparison. Gone are the days of going up and down subway stairs, standing on congested train platforms, navigating through crowds at Penn Station to board the LIRR at rush hour, walking through packed LIRR railroad cars to search for a seat, being subject to the almost daily delays or standing inside a stinky elevator. Finding the Express Bus service has provided me with a truly great "workaround" to ease the daily commuting grind. It has made it possible for me to "get out there" and remain an active member of the workforce.

Making a sandwich to take for lunch the next day. Toward the end of the day on Sundays, Mondays, Tuesdays (and sometimes on Wednesdays) after dinner, I will venture to the refrigerator and assorted drawers in the kitchen to assemble things to make a sandwich to pack and bring to work for lunch the next day. Since I generally only go into the city on the first three or four days of the workweek (Monday, Tuesday, Wednesday and sometimes Thursday), I get to take a "sandwich making vacation" the rest of the week. Now preparing lunch for the next workday may seem like a fast and simple task to most people. However, for me it creates extreme difficulty especially since it is a task that I perform at the end of the day when I am most fatigued. I can honestly say that I hate doing this! Early on when I was first diagnosed with MS, making a sandwich for lunch was something I would rush to do in the mornings after eating breakfast and before running out the door. I never even thought about doing this the night before. Nowadays "rushing" and "running" are sports which I have officially retired from, at least for the time being.

Granted this should be a relatively simple process: Grab sandwich meats and mayonnaise/other condiments from the refrigerator, walk over to one of the kitchen cabinets to get wax paper or aluminum foil to wrap the made sandwich in, find a brown paper bag from the cabinet under the kitchen sink, pull out a sandwich roll or sliced bread from one of the kitchen cabinets or the refrigerator, and take a knife from one of the cutlery drawers to help with spreading the mayo onto the bread or roll. When that's all done I then sit on one of the counter stools to prepare and wrap my sandwich. When finished, I wrap the sandwich that I made in aluminum foil and place it into a brown paper lunch bag. I then take the bag, along with the unused cold cuts, mayo and other condiments and put them back into the refrigerator. I toss any garbage into the trash and wash any utensils used in the preparation process. Simple, right? Well, for most people this is a mindless three-minute activity. For someone having MS like me this becomes at a ten minute plus dreaded chore. It gets worse when I drop something on the floor or if I cannot find everything I need in its rightful place in the kitchen cabinets, or remember that I forgot to put napkins inside the bag and must walk back to the other side of the kitchen island cabinet to get them. Yes, there are things I have done to make my sandwich making chores easier (like combining some of the things I use into the same kitchen cabinet or drawer, etc.). But in general there is no "workaround" for this. I will not ask for Luisa's help, as she would generally sit in the den after dinner with Deanna and Lauren (when they both lived at home) to relax and watch television. I do not want to interrupt and bother her, especially after she has prepared dinner. On occasion when I am just too tired, I will not prepare anything the night before and will instead buy a sandwich from the delicatessen which is located downstairs – just a short walk away from my office.

<u>Making the bed.</u> On weekend mornings since I do not go into my office in the city, I try my best to make the bed and save Luisa the trouble of doing so. Up until 2013, I would do this seemingly easy chore most Saturdays and Sundays when I had the "uuummmpp-phhh" to do so. What normally would be less than a two minute exercise would take me about five minutes. Some days it took me longer than that, but I persevered. As time went on it became more challenging for me to navigate from one side of the bed to the other, tuck in the sheets and blankets and grab the throw pillows atop the dresser and place them on the bed. There were days however that I just felt like I could not do it, so I would not. But there were other days that I pushed myself to make the bed and give Luisa a small break. This was one less thing for her to do. And on some days while I had every intention of doing the deed, I just could not. So I would leave the bed unmade and hobble into the kitchen clutching my cane to grab breakfast. On occasion I still face the challenge "head on" when I'm feeling "off" and tidy up the bedroom as best I can. If I have even the slightest bit of energy, I push myself. Ten years prior I would have never even imagined I'd be giving making the bed a second thought. Who knew!

<u>Getting the decorations down from the attic at Christmas time and trimming the tree.</u> Since I began traveling for work in the early 1980s, I started the tradition of buying a Christmas ornament from each place that I visited. As I have traveled to nearly forty-five states

and multiple cities within them as well having traveled to Europe and Asia, I have been able to amass quite a collection of "special" ornaments. Add to that the ornaments Luisa and I have picked-up from the nearly annual vacations we have gone on since the time we were married in 1984 (mostly to Europe and a number of Caribbean islands), plus the souvenirs and gifts many of our friends and family have given to us over the years when they became aware that we were "Christmas ornament junkies." I'd venture to guess that we have more than two-hundred unique Christmas ornaments neatly stored in boxes in the attic. Each one of them tells a story, kind of neat! Each December I would make the annual "pilgrimage" to the attic and bring down the many boxes of ornaments, the artificial Christmas tree, lights and other assorted holiday trinkets to decorate the house. Luisa would usually help me bring the items down from the attic, and Deanna and Lauren when they lived at home would help too with decorating when they were younger. After stringing lights on the shrubs and railings outside the house, we would come inside and decorate the tree. This was always one of my favorite things to do. Hanging each ornament gave me time to reminisce. It would always bring back many memories, particularly since most of the ornaments were inscribed with dates when we purchased or received them. Taking trips down "memory lane" with each ornament we hung definitely elongated the process, but it was fun. As the years went by I remained adamant about hanging every last ornament on the tree. This was despite Luisa's constant reminders that "what goes up must come down." We dreaded the month of January as it was then time to remove the ornaments from the tree, box them, take down the tree and the lights, pack away the decorations strung throughout the house and bring everything back up to the attic for neat storage until the next year. It was no coincidence that I would have to work late every night and on weekends throughout the month of January (my "work" avoidance scheme)! And without fail as the years went by, Luisa would not resist saying, "See, I told you *not* to take everything down from the attic. It's not easy taking stuff down and it certainly isn't any easier bringing it back up." I would always tell her, "Don't worry, I'll bring them down and will take them back up"… until about 2010.

Around that time my MS symptoms were no longer invisible and pulling down the attic stairs, unpacking and packing up the boxes with the ornaments, carrying the boxes down from and bringing them up to the attic, etc., was something I could no longer do. Granted for a number of years after I was diagnosed, I would sneak up to the attic when no one was at home. I would then carry down a box or two, hang more special ornaments on the tree (hanging them got increasingly more difficult though), bring the empty boxes back up to the attic before anyone came home, take down another box or two, decorate the tree, etc. I would then repeat the process. I did this for another two or three years until I no longer could. Today Luisa (and if the girls are home) will help; but by and large though, she is the one solely responsible for fetching the tree and the ornaments from the attic, doing the decorating, then, taking down the tree, boxing and storing the ornaments. And now Luisa, and not me, is solely responsible for decorating the exterior of the house with lights, but now only minimally. I am truly grateful for her efforts but silently think to myself…, "Gee, I don't see the ornament I got from Singapore," or "I don't see the telephone booth ornament I got from London," or "I wonder what happened to the cactus ornament I got from Arizona." I remember one time asking, "Where is the *xyz* ornament?" and getting a very cold and curt response from Luisa. This was the *first and the last time* that I ever made a comment or asked where an ornament was.

Now at Christmas time I'm just thankful the tree is up and we have a good number of our special ornaments hanging from it. As for the other special ornaments that are not on the tree, they will just have to remain for now tucked away in boxes and stored up in the attic. When the MS "cure" comes I will certainly be sure to bring them down and will personally hang them all on the tree. I can't wait! The good news is that by then when Christmas time comes, I will be able to take the tree and the ornaments down and bring them up to the attic for storage—*ALL BY MYSELF!*

"Relaxing" in the Hamptons: It has been fifteen years since Luisa and I built our second home in East Hampton in 2001. Interesting how things have changed since that time. Today there is no longer any lawn vacuuming, leaf raking or tree pruning going on, by us anyway. Instead of going out to the house each weekend and puttering around every room, weeding the beds outside in the garden, organizing things in the garage or basement, etc., my time out east (which is mostly in the summertime) is now generally spent sitting out back or relaxing on a mesh float in the cool pool water. Rarely now do I "get lost for hours" in the basement or in the garage arranging and organizing things. Instead, I watch helplessly as Luisa goes from room to room vacuuming and cleaning. Around 2015 things started to get more difficult for me. Our house in the Hamptons is about forty-two hundred square feet, about twice the size of our primary residence in Jericho. Compared to the house in Jericho, this two-story house in the Hamptons is quite expansive. The rooms are larger and the open floor plan makes getting around more of a challenge for me. "Wall walking" is now more difficult too since the rooms are larger and the walls are farther apart. Since the master bedroom, den, living room and kitchen are on the main level, I now very seldom have a need to go up to the second floor even though

241

the loft there serves as a semi-office. I generally bring a laptop computer to the house, sit downstairs and connect to the wireless internet. As such there is really not much of a reason at all for me to go upstairs to the loft and access the internet via the desktop computer.

There are many small and simple everyday tasks that are just not that easy for me to do anymore. Things like changing the battery of a wall clock, or replacing a light bulb in a ceiling high-hat, or cleaning a spill on the kitchen floor, or squeegeeing the shower after using it, or hanging the American flag outside in the front of the house for holidays like Memorial Day, July 4th and Labor Day, or fixing the closet door that occasionally comes off the track in the laundry room, or helping to fold the laundry after it comes out of the clothes dryer, or wiping down fingerprint smudges on the French glass doors that line the back of the house, etc.: these things are just not that simple for me to do any longer. I now sit on the sidelines and observe, as my wife does most of the things that I once did. I'm frustrated, have a sense of powerlessness and feel somewhat guilty. These feelings have become further amplified as I sometimes hear Luisa breathe a heavy sigh, or mumble under her breath as she undertakes a simple "fix-it" project or takes-on a normal household task. Generally she does this when she thinks I'm not within hearing distance. But I'm sensitive to this and hear things. At times though, Luisa directly voices her frustrations and tells me straight out that she cannot do it anymore and recommends that we sell the house. One can only imagine how lousy this makes me feel. Other times however, things seem okay. As much as she'd never admit it, I actually believe that Luisa likes doing/fixing things and puttering around the house. On occasion out of frustration, Luisa will blurt out, "Let's just sell this place." I often think that Luisa might be right and that selling the house may be the best thing. However, I remain adamant and respond to her that parting with the house is not something I wish to even consider. "Sell our dream house in the Hamptons that we built? No way," I think to myself. However there is no escaping the fact that most, if not all of the upkeep for the house now falls upon Luisa's shoulders and I am just a passive bystander. Thank you, MS! Like many things in my life where I was able to figure out workarounds or improvise to make things a bit easier, the truth of the matter is that there are just some simple everyday things that, when it comes to owning a home (let alone owning a second home out on the east end of Long Island), that I have difficulty doing.

Let's face it, the upkeep associated with owning a home is a lot of work for any healthy person. Factor in a person having a disabling disease like MS and it only becomes increasingly more difficult to maintain things in a consistent manner. I have become victim to this horrible disease and I struggle with my desire to keep the house and balance this with the reality that Luisa is the point-person largely responsible for our home's upkeep. She is truly the 'superintendent' of our second home in the Hamptons (and for that matter, the 'superintendent' for our primary residence in Jericho too)! Sell the house or keep it: This is a balancing act that I think about and face every day. I constantly remind myself that the "super" (Luisa) can only do so much!

Looking for something that has not been returned to its rightful place: Something that has always driven me crazy (and still does) is my inability to find something because it has not been returned to its proper place. Whether it be a screwdriver or a hammer, a garden shovel or a rake, the cordless electric drill or its bits, a pair of reading magnifier glasses, the cordless telephone, a scotch tape dispenser or a pair of scissors, the television remote control, etc. As a prefectionist and a highly organized sole, I have always gone to great lengths to store and organize things in a very logical and orderly fashion. For example, I recall putting up peg boards in our garage many years ago when we first built the house to better organize and find household tools when they were needed, and having a place to return them. This worked nicely for a while but it seemed that as time went by, tools that were removed from their spot on the peg boards never seemed to make it back from where they came from. The perception that I was a highly organized stickler was one that always preceded me. For example, people that I worked with over twenty years ago would frequently tease me and ask if I indexed the food I stored in my kitchen pantry cabinets, or color coded the clothes hanging in my by bedroom closets, or alphabetized by brand the cereal boxes I kept in my kitchen cupboards, etc.

Many years before I was diagnosed with MS and did not even have a clue what it was, I was always the one who would organize things like tools, pick up items that were left behind by others and return them to their "assigned" place, organize papers, etc. This became more or less of a habit for me. In fact, I was happy to pick things up. Many times I would look for a certain tool or other item in its "assigned" place and because I couldn't find it, I would make a trip to the garden center or the hardware store to buy it again. Then several months later, the item would "turn up" and we'd have two of them. In my pre-MS days, I was able to shrug this off and had no problem with things not being returned to their rightful place. I chalked this up to "that's just the way things are" and seldomly complained.

Yes, I'm frustrated. For example I would become increasingly more frustrated whenever I'd look for an item to use (like a stapler or reading glasses or a Philips screwdriver, etc.) and it is not where it "should be." As time went by, my tolerance level for becoming annoyed began to increase. It was tough "getting up" off the couch and searching for a pair of scissors or magnifying readers, or getting up to answer a ringing telephone that I could not find because it had not been returned to its charging cradle, etc. Yes, these things annoyed me and searching for them became increasingly more difficult for me to do. Because Luisa was always the one fixing things around the house due to my inability to do so, as time went on I learned not to voice my frustrations. Many times I just bite my lip and do not say a word. So I'd wind up buying things that I frequently used in the past but could no longer find (i.e. like reading glasses, scissors, tape dispensers, etc.) and "hide" them from Luisa by placing them in obscure places (i.e. like under the couch in the den or in the far corner of a drawer in a kitchen cabinet, etc.). I place these items in "hidden alcoves" that only I knew about and could easily access. Thank goodness for my frequent "Target runs" so that I can easily re-purchase items that I cannot find that need to be replenished. Today, I just move forward and seldom say anything. Yes, it is very annoying, but I've learned to accept this and move on. At one point we'll likely need to have a garage sale so we can rid ourselves of all of the duplicate tools and office supplies that are likely to turn up in the house down the road!

Installing a remote-control thermostat in the house: During the summer and winter months, Luisa and I usually play "dueling thermostats." In the summertime I prefer and need it to be cool in the house so I will typically turn the thermostat down to seventy/seventy-one degrees so the air conditioning kicks on more frequently. Located in the hallway just outside the master bedroom of our home in Jericho, almost every time I walk past the thermostat I notice that it has miraculously been reset to seventy-four degrees, if not higher. So the next time I walk by the thermostat I turn it down once more. Later on I notice the thermostat has again been reset. This goes on almost continuously. During the winter months, the opposite occurs. I turn the thermostat down when the house is hot so the heat shuts off, and Luisa turns it up. She says that she feels cold and raises the thermostat in order to turn up the heat.

Today I have since found a way to discretely adjust the settings to a more comfortable and suitable level for me. I have had installed a wireless remote-controlled thermostat—the Nest. This allows me to re-set the temperature remotely from my cell phone. With the Nest, not only do I save myself the trouble of getting-up and walking (limping) over to reset the thermostat, I can now do it (unbeknownst to Luisa) after she falls asleep. And I can reset the temperature when I am out of the house and on my way home so that by the time I arrive home, the house is at a comfortable temperature. The end result: A more comfortable and suitable temperature that allows me to function somewhat normally. Take that, MS!!

• • • • •

All things considered though, I can't help but think that my situation could be a lot worse. The modifications I that I *have* been able to make, the workarounds that I *have* adopted and the tolerances that I *have* built to deal with my frustrations have all allowed me to maintain a fairly "normal" lifestyle, or so I think. Fatigue is one of the biggest issues which I now face, particularly toward the end of most days. It doesn't hit me every day, but when it does—I know it. On these days all I want to do is get off my feet and relax. Luckily it's usually an end-of-the day phenomenon, so around 8 P.M. or 9 P.M. each evening I'm getting set to relax and unwind anyway. Lying down in bed at that time of day to read or watch television isn't so bad. According to the National Multiple Sclerosis Society, 80 percent of people with MS suffer from fatigue. MS-related fatigue tends to get worse as the day goes on, so I guess I'm"normal" in this regard. It is often aggravated by heat and humidity, so thank goodness my home has central air conditioning. MS related fatigue comes on more easily and suddenly than normal fatigue. Balance is another factor that often comes into play and my struggles to maintain a steady state take a lot out of me. I guess that struggling some days to maintain my equilibrium and stressing out about it makes my body work harder, thereby further adding to my fatigue. This seems logical to me. However there is no scientific medical evidence that supports this premise, or as I like to refer to it as "The Spoto Hypothesis."

The true cause of fatigue in MS remains largely unknown. However, the likely causes are structural abnormalities in the brain caused by demyelination and axonal loss. This can be attributed to immune activity in the brain itself, problems of hormone production from the pituitary gland in the brain or due to problems with chemical changes in the muscles. Someone at an MS conference once told me that MS fatigue comes about due to the fact that the body needs to work harder in order to transmit signals from the brain since areas of demyelination frequently disrupt the transmission path and make the sending of signals a more arduous task. Since brain signals escape in the demyelinated "wires" that carry them, the body needs to work (or push) harder to transmit signals to the targeted endpoints. This sounds logical and makes perfect sense to me, and only provides more logic to support the "Spoto Hypothesis."

I generally keep my fatigue to myself and will rarely say anything to anyone, including Luisa. After all, most times she has generally had a hard day too. I understand that Luisa is also tired, so I rarely mention anything anymore about me being tired. On occasion I will blurt out the fact that I am tired and am going to lie down. I do not do this to evoke pity or sympathy, but rather it just comes out of my mouth spontaneously.

I'm counting down the time until scientists and researchers find something to help restore functionality that has either been lost or compromised by MS, a "cure" some might say. Until that day, I will keep a positive mindset and try to find creative ways to develop workarounds to do things, and deal with my "end-of-day" fatigue. I often think to myself: "Limitations, what do you mean? What limitations?"

Chapter 13

The Chore of Walking

There are some everyday things in life which are so common and ordinary that you just take them for granted. That is until you can no longer do them *or* until you can no longer do them as *effortlessly* as you once did. Walking is one such thing.

It wasn't until several years after my diagnosis in 2006 and I began to experience foot drop that I started to have walking issues. At first it was as simple as not being able to keep up with others or walking with a slight limp or feeling fatigued when I walked longer distances. The good news was that I had maybe one or two stumbles and may have tripped only once or twice during this time, but nothing that resulted in any injuries that I was unable to quickly recover from that kept me from resuming my *normal* activities. I was generally able to mask my walking challenges and come up with excuses for my limp that I would tell others as need be. As time went on and my foot drop became more pronounced, it became increasingly more difficult for me to walk normally and keep up with others. I would swing my left leg out to the side and walk with a prominent limp. After a while I got fitted for a foot brace to help improve my overall stability; this allowed me to reduce the degree of foot drop that I was experiencing and walk a little faster. That lasted for a little less than one year, and later on I purchased and got fitted for an electronic stimulation device (which I discuss in detail in an earlier chapter). I purchased a device called the Bioness L300 in the hopes that it could provide added benefit. For a while it did, or so I thought. At one point I finally gave in and had to start using a cane to help me walk and maintain my balance; I continue to use a cane to this day. Throughout this entire time and through the present, I'd walk "peg-legged." My left leg is almost totally stiff and I am currently unable to bend my knee when walking. I continue to throw my leg out to the side with each step that I take. Doing the normal "heal-then-toe" walking routine has become increasingly more difficult for me, something I try doing today but am at most times unable to. To complicate matters more, my balance has become worse thereby contributing further to my walking challenges. I just hope I never get pulled over by a police officer and am asked to walk a straight line for sobriety testing purposes!

Fear of falling, something I never even thought of before, is constantly on my mind now. As such this fear of falling has made walking a more planned and deliberate activity for me. When I walk from the bus stop to my office in Manhattan, I am cautious and make sure I remain far away from the curb and the street just in case I lose my balance and fall. I don't want to wind up falling in the roadway and getting hit by a car or a bus! There are some days when I choose not to get up and walk around my home or my office, unless I absolutely have to. It is easy to succumb to this and remain idle, but I do my best to "not give in" and will always push myself and get up and walk unless I'm having a really bad day. Walking has become even more of a challenge for me in the warmer, summer months as the heat further contributes to my unbalanced and "wobbly" state. I've gotten somewhat used to walking "peg-legged," and now officially define walking as a challenge. Walking is a common everyday thing which I wish I did not have to think about.

But I do. Thank goodness for walls, as "wall-walking" has become a common practice for me particularly when moving from room to room inside my house. (Subsequently in early 2016, I 'gave-in' and purchased a three wheel 'rollator' or walker which I bring with me on the bus into Manhattan when I commute). The unit, which is made of lightweight aluminum, weighs all of about seven pounds and folds quickly into a neat and portable device, has been a godsend and quite honestly is something I cannot imagine having done without previously. It has also given me more confidence to take short walks from my office onto the street below to visit nearby delicatessens and convenience stores - when the weather permits.

Toward the end of 2013, my balance began to worsen even more. As a result I was feeling less stable whenever I walked. I became particularly challenged when walking down stairs or navigating down even the slightest incline. Walking in crowded places like Penn Station or a shopping mall presents big problems for me too, so I continue to avoid this. Walking along the beach or even on a soft grassy surface in a park or lawn is something I can no longer easily do either, even with my cane. When I walk along the sidewalk and come to a corner, I have difficulty stepping off the curb to cross the street. Nowadays most street corners in Manhattan have sidewalk squares with gradual downward slopes leaning toward the street that are designed to make crossing somewhat easier for handicap people using wheelchairs and other assisted devices. However, certain street corners in Manhattan have sloped concrete squares in which the downward slants are anything but gradual. Some of these sloped concrete squares contain steep angles that make stepping down them and crossing the street a problem for me. So today I take my time when walking and crossing any street to prevent myself from falling. There was a point in time that I looked forward to the end of each work day, packing up my belongings and walking to the subway or to Penn Station in order to board the rail road to my home on Long Island. However, over the last few years I have come to dread the end of the work day knowing that I need to leave the office and get up and walk. Granted, taking the Express Bus means having to walk less than I did previously when I was taking the rail road out of Penn Station. But it still means that I have to walk, something so natural that I *never* even gave any thought to doing—until around 2012.

Sometime in mid-2014 the enterprise operating the Express Bus service into Manhattan (Go Buses) was sold to another company (Academy). With my office just off 6th Avenue on 45th Street, I was fortunate up until this time that drivers of the Express Bus, which turned onto 6th Avenue from 34th Street after exiting the midtown tunnel and travelling uptown, made a special accommodation for me by making an unscheduled stop that I requested each morning on the corner of 45th Street and 6th Avenue. Since I began commuting into midtown I basically had the same morning driver, Ray who always made this special accommodation stop for me. The regularly scheduled bus stops were on 42nd and 6th and 48th and 6th, so the courtesy stop on 45th each morning was a great help in that it saved me from walking three blocks (not any big deal for most people, but a HUGE deal for me). In the evenings I would walk to the bus stop on 42nd Street and 6th Avenue. That extra three block walk in the evening was a given, and there really wasn't anything I could do about that. I remember that my walk each evening when I first started taking the midtown Express Bus would take me just under ten minutes to go the three-plus blocks. I would depart my office around 5:10 P.M. and make it to the bus stop comfortably by the 5:20 P.M. pick-up time. I remember counting the steps I took within each concrete square or flag (why I counted them, I'll never know). Initially, it took me about two steps to walk across each concrete flag. As time went on and about two-plus years later, my four block/ten-minute walk in the evenings would take me almost twenty minutes, and my steps within each sidewalk concrete flag went from two to almost three.

Starting some time during 2013 I began to leave my office about ten minutes earlier, or no later than 4:55 P.M. in order to make it in time for the 5:20 P.M. Express Bus pick-up. I was pooped by the time I got to the bus stop on 42nd Street and 6th Avenue. Leaving the office a few minutes earlier each afternoon helped ensure I made it to the bus stop on time. Funny thing, as fate would have it there were always three hard plastic milk crates chained to the lamp post by the 42nd Street bus stop. Whenever I approached the bus stop I'd plop myself down on the crates. They became my makeshift "bench," which I was very happy to have. At first I figured the milk crates would only be there temporarily. Each morning when the bus would pass by 42nd Street I'd glance out the window and would notice that the milk crates were not there. However, by day's end they were back and were chained to the same lamp post. They must have belonged to a street vendor or to someone who would store and chain them to the lamp post at the end of each day so they could retrieve them the next morning. Whatever the case, I was not about to complain. This makeshift "bench" was around for over one year until I no longer needed it due to the eventual addition of a new bus stop (which I talk about below) on the corner of my office on 45th Street and 6th Avenue.

After the bus company was sold to Academy, an entirely new crew of drivers was hired. This new group of bus drivers were instructed by the company to adhere only to the scheduled stops; no special stops or courtesy accommodations would be made—period. Unlike with the previous company where more or less the same drivers drove each day, the drivers hired by Academy changed almost daily and there was little if any continuity. For the first few weeks after the ownership change I would kindly ask each driver on my morning commute before approaching 45th Street (from the front seat of the bus where I sat) if they would be kind enough to do a courtesy stop for me on the on the corner of 45th Street. The majority of the time, the drivers said, "No, sorry," they could not make any unscheduled stops. On rare occasions a driver would in fact accommodate me. I was surprised that as time went on, many of my fellow commuters became quite vocal and pressed the drivers that wouldn't accommodate me as to the reason why they would not. On some days the dialogues my fellow passengers had with the bus drivers became quite heated, especially with one driver who was actually one of the few who consistently did the morning run a couple of times per week. To put it mildly, this driver was downright nasty each time I would politely ask him if he'd stop. On a few occasions some of my fellow commuters got into shouting matches with him. I felt so embarrassed, and recall one day when a fellow passenger came to my defense and shouted at the bus driver, "If it were your mother, would you stop?" The bus driver and my fellow commuter quickly exchanged words, with the bus driver screaming back, "You leave my mother out of this!" I was mortified. Thank you, MS!

I later learned that several of my other fellow commuters called the corporate office on my behalf. Feeling very humbled by their support, I was again somewhat embarrassed. They also continued arguing almost daily with the drivers to make a special stop in order to accommodate me. I do not think that any of my commuters who argued on my behalf knew I had MS. I never told anyone. They just saw that I walked with a cane and correctly assumed that I was a special needs person with some type of disability who required assistance. Perhaps some of them may have had an inkling that I may have had MS, but they never asked. And, I never volunteered the information.

As the weeks went by several of my fellow commuters would tell me almost daily that I should contact the bus company and request that a formal stop be added on 45th and 6th, both in the mornings *and* in the evenings. Initially I shrugged off that idea and remained adamant about not wanting to request any special treatment. The more I thought about it though the more inclined I became to call the bus company and request that the additional afternoon stop be added. Then one night the straw that broke the camel's back happened. It was pouring rain as I walked to the 42nd Street bus stop; carrying an umbrella was out of the question, since I held my cane in one hand and wheeled my roller brief case with the other in order to maintain my balance. So by the time I reached the bus stop I was soaking wet. Sitting on the milk crates or on my makeshift 'bench' in the pouring rain made me water logged. To boot, the bus arrived about ten minutes late that particular evening! I was soaked! That did it. Finally, I decided to contact the bus company's corporate headquarters. Yes I gave-in and figured 'special treatment' may not be so bad after all. The next day I placed a call into the CEO's office at Academy and left a voice message. I also followed-up with an email and a letter which I physically mailed. About two weeks went by and I did not get any response. Like I did previously when I contacted the CEO's office at the exercise facility voicing concerns about the absence of a handicap ramp, I followed-up with another phone call and email expressing my disdain with their lack of professionalism in at least acknowledging and responding to my prior communications. Below is the email that I sent to the Academy bus company:

My name is Vincent Spoto. I am a special needs person with an impaired gait due to my having Multiple Sclerosis. While I am ambulatory, I do walk with the assistance of a cane. I currently commute from Christopher Morley Park in Manhasset Long Island to midtown Manhattan generally 3 to 4 days per week, and have been doing so for approximately 4 years

Currently, I work on 45th Street off 6th Avenue. Two of the official bus stops for the midtown run are: (i) on 6th Avenue and 42nd Street, and (ii) on 6th Avenue & 48th Street.

Since I have been riding the bus and prior to Academy taking over from the previous owners (Go Buses), each and every bus driver (and there have been close to a half dozen of them over past several years) has made a courtesy stop for me on the southeast corner of 6ᵗʰ Avenue and 45ᵗʰ Street. They did this as a special needs accommodation, with me nicely asking the bus driver for a favor on the bus each day and without having to reach out to corporate headquarters for specific approval.

Since the sale of the company to Academy, the drivers have been unwilling to do this. They site liability concerns and have advised me to speak with the corporate office to see if an official stop on 45ᵗʰ Street and 6ᵗʰ Avenue can be designated or if an formal stop, at least in the mornings, can be made for my situation.

Funny, because the bus passes 45ᵗʰ Street anyway as part of its normal run along 6ᵗʰ Avenue, and the majority of the time stops for a red traffic light on that corner anyway.

The drop-offs made for me in the past on 45ᵗʰ & 6ᵗʰ as an accommodation have been <u>extremely</u> helpful, and have enabled me to continue working in Manhattan. The drop-off on the corner of 45ᵗʰ and 6ᵗʰ makes it easier and much less of a challenge for me to navigate the 3 long city blocks necessary when walking to my office from the 'official' stop on 6ᵗʰ Avenue on 42ⁿᵈ Street.

As I have previously written to the company and placed several phone calls into the CEO's office about this matter, I am ex-

tremely disappointed that no one from Academy has had the professional courtesy to at least contact me to discuss this situation. If I do not hear back from anyone in your office within the next two weeks, I will have no choice but to take my story to the newspaper and television outlets and to also register a formal complaint with the appropriate contact at the U.S. Department of Justice responsible for administering the Americans with Disabilities Act (ADA). I remain hopeful that this will not become necessary.

Thank you for your attention to this matter. I look forward to hearing from your office shortly.

Within forty-eight hours of sending this email, the Director of Safety Administration for the Academy bus company called me to apologize and indicate that effective immediately, a morning and an evening stop for the Express Bus midtown run would be added on 45th Street and 6th Avenue, and that if I had any questions or concerns I should feel free to contact him directly. There was no discussion, as apparently my letter was clear and to the point. The gentleman who contacted me was very apologetic that I never received a response. He was extremely kind and freely offered to accommodate me. He gave me both his office and personal cell phone number. There was no need for me to have to explain things any further, as he confirmed my assumption and told me that my letter was self-explanatory and that no further details were required. In early 2015 the company operating the Express Bus service between Long Island and Manhattan was sold yet again, this time from Academy to the North Fork Express. The nice thing was that the North Fork Express company honored the commitment made by Academy, and continued making stops at 45th and 6th both in the mornings and in the evenings.

The addition of this new bus stop made a huge difference for me, and significantly lessened my chore of walking. I no longer had to rely on the milk crates chained to the 42nd Street lamp post that served as my makeshift "bench." It is hard to imagine something as small as an added bus stop that eliminated the need to walk three extra blocks could have such a huge impact, but it did. I was beginning to realize that what my dad constantly said to me growing up was true: "Stand up and fight for yourself always, and don't be afraid to speak-up for something that you feel you deserve. If you don't stand up for yourself, people will walk all over you." I realize now that my father was right. I'm sure he is smiling and very proud of me today as he looks down from heaven.

As much as I hated to admit it, the lack of mobility I was experiencing relating to my walking was becoming quite noticeable to others. No longer did I have a slight or casual limp and no longer was I able to shrug it off by telling others that it was nothing. I guess this came to a head when my business partners, Allen and Brian had a heart-to-heart talk with me. For several months at the end of 2014 our business had slowed temporarily and we were no longer winning jobs with the same degree of frequency as we had in the past. Finally, there was a light shining on the horizon. We were invited to address in person a larger group of lawyers, after having a very successful telephone conference call with a smaller group of attorneys representing the plaintiffs for a case. This initial call went great, and was a preliminary test that that we apparently "passed" with flying colors. We were asked to present once again at a follow-up meeting, this time in person.

The day before we would be presenting, Allen and Brian pulled me aside in the conference room in our office. After engaging in small talk for a few minutes, they told me that it would probably be better if I called into the meeting and did not participate in person. I listened stoically and with a puzzled look on my face asked, "*Why?*" There was a long period of silence that filled the room. Finally, Allen (who did most of the talking) went on to tell me that because this was potentially such a large and lucrative job for RRMS that likely would result in expert witness court testimony, both he and Brian both believed that it was important to eliminate any potential doubt that the "decision makers" at the client may have when considering us for the assignment. Struggles with my gait were obvious, and something I could no longer mask. Allen was very blunt and said that it was obvious I was struggling daily with walking and getting around. He was absolutely right. I was probably in denial, but truth be told walking had become a real chore for me. Allen went on to say that the scheduled in-person presentation for this case was with a larger group of approximately fifteen attorneys and as such, it was unknown as to whether anyone in the room would read into my disability and silently find reason *not* to hire us. Allen immediately then told me that neither he nor Brian felt in any way that my disability had any impact on my cognitive abilities to perform and deliver superior results to the client (which certainly it did not)! Brian then jumped into the discussion adding that while no one else in the room of lawyers would ever admit to being prejudice or biased in any way, there was always a chance that someone could feel that our ability to do the job may be compromised, especially since the engagement would likely require travel to the client's sites in Florida and Texas. "Perception is reality," Brian said, "and let's face it, some people are ignorant." He was right. I nodded and told him that I understood. The goal was to eliminate any potential reason or doubt for not hiring RRMS for this assignment. Allen, Brian and I all shared this belief. Still though, I was upset.

While I was not at all happy with the situation, I truly did understand. I knew that this must have been a very difficult discussion for both Allen and Brian to have with me. However, it was equally as difficult for *me* to listen to it. Rather than sulk and argue, I accepted their decision and we agreed that I'd participate in the meeting via a conference call. Apparently there were a few out-of-state lawyers that would also be dialing into the meeting anyway, so I would not be the only person participating remotely. Silently I began to doubt my worth, but I persevered. By participating via phone no one would see me hobble into the room with my cane, thereby eliminating the possibility that anybody may have secretly said to themselves, *"Hey, what's wrong with this guy. One of the top three guys in this firm has difficulty walking, keeping his balance and standing? One of the founding partners, no-less? Do we really want to hire a firm where one third of the senior management team appears to be 'lame'? If this case ever goes to court, would he ever be able to testify as an expert witness?"*

Again, Allen and Brian both pointed out that no one would ever dare to ask such questions aloud. However, no one could control what people may have thought silently and could potentially use as an excuse for not hiring RRMS. It was the end of the day anyway, so I had plenty of time to think and reflect on what Allen and Brian had told me. I left the office and made my new-found half a block short pilgrimage to the bus stop on 45th and 6th. To put it bluntly, I was pissed—not at Allen and Brian, but at *me*; at *me* for having this dreadful disease and it having such a real and noticeable impact on my mobility. And I was very disappointed about the reality that was setting in that my disability was beginning to have an impact on my business, RRMS Advisors. I was saddened, frustrated and upset. I was really pissed off! Being told that it may be in the best interest of the business for me *not* to attend the meeting in person was devastating! But I somehow understood and after stepping back, I let my emotions subside and had some time to reflect. I knew that what Allen and Brian were saying made perfect sense. After all, winning business was a common goal that we all shared and making money was our biggest priority. Besides, like Allen and Brian would always tell me, they believed that my having MS in no way interfered with my cognitive abilities that were necessary in order for me to deliver superior results to the client!

I went home and shared my frustration and disappointment with Luisa. It felt good to vent. One thing I did know for sure and kept telling myself was that while my mobility may be compromised, my mind and cognitive abilities continue to function at full throttle. As such my ability to reason, communicate verbally with others, think rationally and commit my thoughts to writing was unaffected. Each of these attributes was essential to running my business.

One week later both Allen and Brian attended the client meeting in person and I participated remotely by telephone. The meeting lasted about one hour and went very well. We were asked back the following week as one of the finalists to now meet with the trustees involved, as well as meet with some of the lawyers who also attended the initial meeting. For this third and presumably final meeting, many of the trustees participating were not in the New York area so a webcast video conference was added this time. Like the previous meeting, Allen and Brian participated in person and travelled to the client's office which was only about five blocks from our midtown Manhattan workplace. And like the previous meeting, I participated remotely this time though through a tele-video conference. So, I had to be sure I looked presentable from the waste-up. I wore blue jeans, sported a crisp blue button-down oxford shirt, and donned a red tie and a sport jacket. It would not have even mattered if I wasn't wearing trousers, thanks to today's web-ex technology. But rest assured though, I was wearing pants! Admittedly participating in this meeting remotely was much easier for me to accept than it was when I was asked *not* to participate in-person at the prior meeting held the week earlier. This probably related to the fact that the shock and sadness I experienced when initially told I would not be participating in person had passed. "Lights, camera, and action"—I was now ready to roll!

Meeting with clients and doing business pitches was a critical role which I played for RRMS, partnering with both Allen and Brian in order to help win new business. Plus, preparing marketing pitches and doing presentations was something I really enjoyed doing. And quite frankly it was something I was pretty good at too! I equally enjoyed not only preparing the presentations, but also physically presenting in front of clients. Once we would win new business, we would mostly send contract workers out to the client's site to do much of the legwork anyway. Allen or Brian would fulfill the on-site supervisory role the three of us had as partners. They would travel to the client frequently to "check things out" whenever necessary, and there was rarely a need for me to travel for this. However, on very rare occasions I would. The large majority of the time I would hold conference calls each week from our New York City office with the RRMS supervisors and staff on-site at the client's workplace, just to keep my finger on the pulse as to what was going on. I tended to be "hands-on" anyway, so doing these weekly calls was second nature for me. Additionally I became "anointed" as the RRMS partner to receive, review for accuracy/reasonableness and edit (in some case rewrite) all narrative summaries and preliminary reports that were drafted by our on-site contractors and staff before anything was finalized and given to the client. I guess my undergraduate college degree as an English Writing major had paid-off! Reviewing, editing and re-writing narrative text was starting to morph into a new role for me. It was something I had no choice but to make adjustments for and accept. I didn't mind though, as writing came relatively easy for me and was something I actually enjoyed doing!

Walking and getting around had become more difficult for me, and the simple task of "sauntering about the office" had now officially become a "chore." Allen and Brian were right. The good news was that I was still ambulatory, although now I relied exclusively on my cane to get around. Prior to this point in 2014, I used the cane more or less as the assistive device it was intended to be. It was something that I placed occasional reliance on for support to help me walk on difficult days.

Around 2014 my cane became more of a necessity that I needed every day _to_ help me walk and maintain my balance.

Sadly, the wind up was that we did _not_ win the job and lost it to one of our competitors. I guess Allen and Brian did what they thought was best when they decided and convinced me _not_ to participate in person. Obviously my attending or not attending in person had no bearing on the final outcome and the decision made regarding RRMS not winning the engagement. Who knows though, had I attended in person one of the attorneys may have so enamored by my presence and good looks that we may have been awarded the assignment instantaneously. Hahahaha!

A few weeks later, another engagement opportunity presented itself. We were asked to fly out to California as one of the finalists for a third-party consultant/advisory audit servicing surveillance job that we had applied for several months earlier. Landing this assignment was clearly a long-shot. It paid substantially and was scheduled to last a minimum of twenty-four months. Since RRMS was relatively small in size (especially with respect to net worth and total sales when compared with other companies, like the big four accounting firms who were our likely competitors), the possibility of winning the job seemed somewhat remote. Nonetheless though out of approximately fifty firms who initially applied for the assignment, we were one of seven finalists selected and invited out to California to present. Not bad! We literally had one week to pull together a detailed presentation to make in Sacramento, California to the state commissioner responsible for business oversight. So for five straight days I went into presentation mode. I wrote about a subject that was directly in my wheelhouse—residential mortgage loan servicing surveillance and oversight. About two days before the scheduled presentation date in California, I sat down with Allen and Brian once again. Only this time they told me they were concerned with my health and thought it was probably in my best interest _not_ to fly out to Sacramento for the presentation, especially since we would be returning back to New York on a red-eye flight later in the day that we were scheduled to present. Both Allen and Brian feared that the long flight to the West Coast, coupled with the rush to present and with the scurrying associated with the same-day turnaround by taking the red-eye would create too much stress and anxiety for me to handle. There was no mention by them this time of the negative client perceptions that may have been created by me attending in person, or my limited mobility and the fact that I needed a cane to help me stand upright and walk. Although I'm sure this was in the back of their minds too. Again I was not happy that I would *not* be part of the in-person presentation, but had no rational argument to make about not participating. This one weighed particularly heavy on me though, probably because the subject matter was so complimentary to my experience and skill set. True, I could have argued and made a big stink about going—but I did not. For this presentation, no teleconference or web-ex video would be arranged. So participating remotely was not an option for me. I wished both Allen and Brian the best of luck on the trip to California, and went to the gym that afternoon instead!

When Allen and Brian came back into the office on Monday after traveling to the West Coast, they were both very positive and felt there was a very strong possibility that RRMS would be invited back as one of the two finalists to present and interview for final consideration. Allen was particularly bullish about our chances to win the engagement. However, Brian remained true to form and was a bit more reserved. I was not surprised that things went well, as both Allen and Brian were excellent at presenting and both had strong product knowledge and experience. Plus they had a very strong and well put-together power-point presentation deck that the other RRMS partner who stayed behind in New York had put together. Gee, I wonder who that could have been?

For about one month after these two engagement pitches were made I remained in a funk of sorts, largely due to the fact that I could not help but think that my disability was beginning to have an impact on my business. Being told by my partners that it would be best if I stepped aside and did not present in front of potential clients was devastating! The truth of the matter though was that I indeed had difficulties walking, with some days being worse than others. Walking had become a real chore that I did not want to deal with. At one point I really had to push myself to leave the house to even go into the office, or go to the gym, or visit my father, or see my trainer, or run errands, etc. But I did push myself and as a result, my work-related "funk" was temporary and pretty short-lived! I kept reminding myself that this MS thing was only temporary and that at some point in the future a cure would be found. Therefore it was absolutely critical that I be fit and fully able to take advantage of it. So there was no room for self-pity. Remaining in a "funk" for any extended period of time was not an option—it was out of the question!

At one point, Brian had offered to give me some complimentary tickets he received from his wife's employer to an upcoming ballgame at Yankee Stadium. I loved seeing the Yankees compete in person and going to the stadium to watch them play. This was something I did with my dad growing up as a little boy, and always got goose bumps every time I walked inside the stadium. Back then my dad would "splurge" for the $2.75 general admission tickets, but would never even think about going for the most expensive seats in the house: The field level box seats which sold at that time for a whopping $4.00 per ticket! And whenever we would go to a ballgame, our general admission seats were inevitably right smack behind one of the steel poles used to support the upper deck that were omnipresent throughout the old stadium. Around 2009 I stopped going to the ballpark, as getting there and navigating around became just too much of a hassle. Plus, forty-plus years later those "top-end" $4.00 field level box seats were now priced at $275.00

(a 6,000 percent+ increase), parking went from $2.00 to $35.00, and the Triboro bridge toll (one-way) rose from .50 cents to $6.50. And did I mention that ballpark hot dogs sold for six dollars versus the 1974 price of fifty cents? Not only was going to the ballpark expensive, it was very tiresome for me and also placed too much of a burden and inconvenience on those who accompanied me. Thank you, MS!

It was just easier and a lot less expensive for me to watch the games on television from the comfort of my own living room. That all changed though in early 2015 when I took Brian up on his offer and accepted the tickets to the Yankee game. As an added bonus, it was a Sunday night game and the Yankees were playing the New York Mets! How could I decline these tickets to the "subway series?"

I had not been to a ball game at Yankee Stadium in six years and I was reluctant to go this time. I knew that the chore of walking awaited me. The day before the game I did phone the stadium's Disability Services Department and explained my situation to them. I had heard that stadium personnel were extremely courteous and accommodating in dealing with patrons having special needs. My telephone conversation with them confirmed this—they were great! They were extremely helpful and directed me to enter the stadium via a special gate and was instructed to visit a Guest Relations area that would exchange my tickets for specially designated handicap seats. They also directed me to a parking garage across the street from the stadium and adjacent to the gate which I was advised to enter so that my walking distance to the ball park would be significantly reduced. Once I arrived at the Yankee Stadium and while at the Guest Relations window, stadium personnel went out of their way to accommodate me. They directed me, Luisa, my daughter Lauren and her friend to a disabled person's seating section very close to the seating area appearing on the tickets given to us by Brian. The seats were outstanding. They were located on the main level of the stadium between home plate and third base. With these seats there was no need to navigate any stairwells or walkways, as the concession stands and restrooms were directly behind us. The seats also offered an unobstructed view of the playing field and were positioned underneath a slight over hang to protect against any inclement weather and also act as a shield from the wind. (I do remember though that it was beautiful that night, just a little crisp and windy). And being slightly beneath an overhang we were shielded from the cold wind that whipped around the playing field, unlike the other patrons at the game who were sitting in the stands.

Seems like the New York Yankees did things right when they built the new stadium in that they allocated a large number of seats around the inside perimeter of the entire main level of the ballpark for individuals having special needs. Wow—other than spending a "week's salary" on parking, the bridge toll, hot dogs and beers I didn't know what I was missing by staying away from the ballpark. The seats were great! Outstanding! I literally did not have to get up to walk anywhere during the entire game, except to the restroom which was a short distance directly behind me. Concierge service was provided with the disability seats, so getting hot dogs and beers was easy and leaving my seat to visit the concession stands was not necessary. The entire experience was relatively hassle free! I was so impressed and happy that I was able to attend the game in-person. It was almost like being reborn! Stadium personnel were extremely professional and very accommodating. They truly helped make my experience quite pleasant and memorable, one which I intend to repeat. This probably seems to others like a small thing, but it actually felt great to get out in a public forum and do something normal! And oh yeah, I also purchased a Yankee yearbook while I was at the game that night for twenty five dollars (versus the 1974 price of fifty cents).

One thing that having MS has taught me is to never give up. Whether it be dealing with issues at work or doing something as simple as going to a ballgame, the key is *not* to give in and *not* to let the enemy win. Granted, it is so much easier to sit back and watch the world go by from the comfort of the couch in your living room. Becoming a "shut-in" is very easy and very tempting to do. Why walk about if you don't have to? It is so easy to just sit back, put your feet up and relax. The key however is to keep fighting, enjoy life and always do what you feel is the right thing. By keeping a positive outlook on life and not wallowing in self-pity, it is much easier to deal with a life-changing event like MS. It is so important to keep doing the everyday things in life that are so common and ordinary that you often take for granted, even though you cannot do them as effortlessly as you once did. Walking is one such thing.

MS teaches you to never take anything for granted and to be thankful for all the simple and basic things that you have in life. Yes, today walking is a chore for me. Seeing people who cannot walk at all or seeing people who are confined to a wheelchair makes me realize how fortunate I am at the present time to be ambulatory and still able to get around to do my "chores."

... And oh, by the way, my firm did not win that California job, which we knew was a long-shot anyway. On to the next one!

Chapter 14

Support Groups and Information Sessions

Growing up as a child, I was never the type of person who embraced the whole concept of joining support groups or attending counseling sessions in order to vet issues and discuss problems. I always believed that people should work out their own issues and not place reliance on psychoanalysis or other types of psychiatric therapies to deal with problems. As such, I never really saw a need to open up and share difficult situations and troubles with uninvolved third-parties. Plus, I'm not afraid to say that I never believed in the whole concept of paying someone to listen to me complain. In my mind the whole concept of seeing a psychiatrist or psychotherapist (or a "shrink" as I used to call them) was something I would always dismiss, as I never believed that therapy sessions did any good. Even after I was initially diagnosed with MS in 2006 and for a number of years afterwards, I remained true to my beliefs. Then around 2012 I began to think differently. The word "shrink" disappeared from my vocabulary, at least when referring to doctors of psychology or psychiatrists. I began meeting others also afflicted with MS and they would frequently speak about some of the benefits they were getting from seeing therapists or participating in group counseling sessions.

As time went on, I began feeling the frustrations that came along with not being able to do the things that I once did. I began noticing that I was becoming short and abrupt at times. Not so much at work or with friends, but more so at home with family. In particular, I would often snap at Luisa and my daughters. Funny because it seemed much easier and more convenient for me to vet my frustrations toward them (my wife in particular)—probably because I knew Luisa was very familiar with my condition and also if nothing more than the mere fact that she was "there." I'm not afraid to admit that I probably took her for granted. Being short and abrupt whenever I would speak occasionally on the telephone with my brothers was not something I would generally do, probably due to the fact that I did not see or talk with them daily, as was the case with my wife. For the most part whenever I spoke with Luisa, I would keep my feelings and anger to myself and would frequently channel my frustrations into short, one-word responses to her questions. A telltale sign that I was frustrated manifested itself in how I'd speak out of the side of my mouth, look down or away, change the subject or act in a totally carefree manner. I meant no disrespect— that's just how I acted. I would also tend to ignore things that were said to me or when I was asked a question; I'd pretend to not hear. I guess that was my way of channeling the frustrations and anger I had when I was having a "bad" day relating to my gait and balance. I'm not ashamed to admit that I still sometimes act this way.

I often wondered how others living with MS handled their frustrations and feelings, so on occasion I would actually take the opportunity to talk with fellow "MS-ers" to find out and satisfy my curiosities firsthand. Eventually, I made meeting with and interacting with others having MS more of a common practice. This has turned out to be, and continues to be, very valuable. As I continued talking more with others, I began to understand and think further about the implications associated with the fact that MS causes demyelination and damage to nerves throughout the *entire* body, including the brain. So logically thinking, if the part of the brain that regulates emotion is damaged, what others told me made sense when they'd say things like such damages often times trigger feelings of anger and depression or anxiety. Researching this matter further, I learned that these feelings often times resulted from a loss of an inhibitory mechanism in the brain that sometimes triggered the release of certain emotions causing moodiness. Also referred to as "emotional liability," the National Multiple Sclerosis Society (NMSS) points out that moodiness can cause a person with MS to experience rapid-fire mood changes; hence, causing them to become "snappy" with a loved one. Even absent any of these neurological factors, living with a chronic and progressive disease in itself can create feelings of anxiety, depression or anger. This, in addition to the scientific factors discussed above, has helped to create the "perfect storm" for me in terms of dealing with life's day-to-day issues. And as much as those close to me try to understand, I really don't think they do.

As much as I hate to admit (and I probably never will, as more often than not I *refuse* to— even to myself), my having MS has perhaps begun to impact my emotional state. I also wonder if MS is responsible for any changes to my cognitive condition as well, only because of something that Deanna, Lauren and (in particular Luisa) often remind me of when it comes to repeating myself: "Yeah, you told me that already," or "this is the third time you've said that." On occasion, they also tell me things (for a second and third time) that they swore they have already mentioned: "I told you this yesterday," or "how many times do I have to tell you the same thing," or "you just choose to conveniently not remember;" these are things that they periodically say to me. I'm not sure if this relates to their lack of any acknowledgment that I said something and therefore say things a second or third time, or if it's because I truly forgot that I previously told them. And there are those very limited occasions where I blurt out a response or statement that appears to be random, out of context or inappropriate. I try not thinking about all this though, as my gait and balance issues always seem to take "center stage" and prohibit me from focusing on anything else. In the back of my mind though, both the moodiness and especially the cognitive piece, are worrisome.

The pharmaceutical companies who make the MS drugs, like Bayer or Biogen or Pfizer, regularly (about once per month) hold information sessions at local restaurants on Long Island, usually providing a complimentary dinner or a boxed lunch. In addition, the makers of Copaxone (Teva Pharmaceuticals), through its network called Shared Solutions, frequently sponsor information sessions as well. Shared Solutions is particularly adept at offering a comprehensive network of free services to help patients with treatment compliance (i.e. adherence to taking the medicine as scheduled, self-injection training, etc.) and ongoing education. Shared Solutions also has a full staff of Teva-trained nurses available twenty-four hours a day to answer questions and provide support. I must say that the companies who manufacture the MS drugs, along with their network affiliates, do an excellent job in working with and educating patients about this dreadful disease. I have found Shared Solutions in particular to be excellent!

Aside from the free food, these information sessions have proven to be a great place to meet people, learn new things and talk with others having MS. Each time I attend a session, I encounter people who share stories about their disability, the day-to-day challenges they face and how they deal with them. At almost every session, I meet new people and learn something that I did not previously know. People I meet seem to always talk about treatments they are receiving, frustrations they have and how they are best coping on a daily basis with having MS. Almost always I meet someone who tells me about an alternative therapy they are trying (like acupuncture, or yoga, or chiropractic), or a food they are consuming (like kale salad, or celery, or horseradish), or a vitamin supplement they are taking (like Calcium, or Ginkgo Biloba, or Turmeric). And most of the time, if the things they talk about sound logical, make sense and are known to *not* have any adverse or contradictory side-effects, I eventually try them out. Applying down my back along my spine a topical cream used to treat athlete's foot and psoriasis (as the cream contains miconazole and clobetasoln, two in-gredients shown to repair nerve fibers in mice that are stripped of myelin), is one of the latest "unconventional" healing remedies that I have learned about and tried. Unfortunately, none of these "remedies" have really worked and made a difference—*yet*, anyway! However, I do plan to keep trying new things; you never know!

Meeting new people almost always results in me getting fresh ideas and perspectives about my disease. This also makes me realize that I am not alone. To my surprise, it amazes me to see how bitter and neg-ative many people suffering with MS are. I guess I understand this, but don't get why people are generally unable (or unwilling) to "dust them-selves off" and move on with life. Don't get me wrong though, for the most part people that I encounter are generally upbeat. Whenever I'm at a table introducing myself and speaking with others, I generally make it a point to be as upbeat and positive as possible, and try my best to lighten the mood. Funny because whenever I speak with others who have MS, I am anything but short and abrupt. This is often times the complete opposite of the way in which I interface with Luisa when dis-cussing my illness. I usually listen attentively to others (so much for the loss of inhibitory mechanisms in the brain triggering the release of emotions that result in feelings of moodiness and depression). Again, this is totally opposite of how I behave when I am around Luisa. I am beginning to realize that the more exposure I have with others who have MS the more comfortable I have begun feeling in my own skin and the more conscious I am becoming of my own actions. Even though I do have MS, I think I have come a long way in not letting my

MS *have me*, and *not* taking my frustrations out on Luisa! At least I try not to! Admittedly though, I still have a ways to go.

Every so often someone that I meet at an information session asks me how I remain so positive and upbeat. Whenever approached with this question, I always smile and say something like, "It is what it is" (I have now learned to hate that tired cliché), or point out that "walking around being angry, negative and complaining is not going to change anything." Typically I will try making a joke to keep things light and upbeat. Aside from meeting and getting to know new people, sharing stories and learning about other alternative therapies and treatments, these sessions are always informative. Most of the time, these gatherings feature talks given by prominent Long Island physicians specializing in MS. On a few occasions, even my neurologist Dr. Blitz has been the featured speaker.

Around 2012, I followed-up on a recommendation provided to me by the Long Island Chapter of the National MS Society and started visiting and spending time talking to a therapist named Jane Elson. Jane specializes in providing counseling services to people having MS. Jane was quite knowledgeable about MS, having spent time previously working as a sales representative for various manufacturers of MS drugs. She also worked with several prominent MS doctors based on Long Island, so she knew their personalities as well as their "hot buttons." Initially, my sessions with Jane were "one-on-one" or private. They provided me with a good outlet to talk about things and air my frustrations. I found it valuable to speak with someone who was not only very knowledgeable about the disease itself, but also someone who had experience dealing with other MS patients and helping them cope with frustrations and issues they encountered on a daily basis. As time went on, Jane formed a Men's Group that initially met twice per month. The group was relatively small and was frequently attended by myself and one other gentleman, Peter. Occasionally, others would attend as well.

These expanded sessions further gave me an opportunity to speak with others having MS and provided me with an opportunity to gain some perspectives about how they were handling the daily challenges they were experiencing. On one occasion, one of the men attending talked about other health issues he had in addition to having MS. I recall this one gentleman in particular, a Gulf War army veteran. He talked not only about his struggles with MS, but also talking about the fact that he was suffering from Post-Traumatic Stress Disorder (PTSD). This was the first time that I ever knowingly met anyone who had PTSD. Listening to his wartime stories reminded me somewhat of listening to my dad when he would tell his accounts of WWII. The biggest difference though is that unlike my dad who seemed to take his experiences in stride and did not emit much emotion about them, this gentleman seemed to get much more emotional and agitated as he went on telling his stories. Perhaps the higher level of emotion he displayed here was related to the fact that this gentleman's wartime experiences occurred relatively recently (i.e. within the past twenty-five years) versus my dad's stories that went back nearly seventy years. One similarity though; both this gentleman and my dad would tell their stories and always remember the most intricate details. Particularly in my dad's case, where the stories went back nearly seven decades, I was quite amazed.

After hearing this and a number of other stories, I realized how fortunate I was that I was not facing another issue aside from, or in addition to, having MS. It became clear to me that having something to deal with beside or in addition to MS could be a hell of a lot worse! In addition to people I'd meet in the Men's Group, often when I was in Jane's office waiting to go into see her or when I was leaving her office after my session was done, I would frequently see and speak with other MS patients who were coming or leaving her office. I really liked going to these sessions held at Jane's office, as (in addition to seeing Jane) they gave me a great opportunity to meet with and talk to others. There were times that I would engage in discussions with people coming and going to the office that lasted longer in duration than the forty-five minute sessions I'd have with Jane. These discussions, along with the time I would spend "one on one" talking with Jane, were invaluable. The more "MS-ers" I spoke with the more I realized that I didn't have things so bad after all.

Peter Licari is close to my age and like me, is fully ambulatory and walks with the assistance of cane (although his gait and balance are slightly better than mine). Peter was diagnosed with MS in 1993, and he actually provided me with the inspiration to write this manuscript. In 1999, Peter published a book about his battle with MS. After reading it I made a decision to become an "author" myself for the first time. Yes, Peter's book inspired me. I only hope that my work is half as good as his!

Similar to me, Peter was an active professional who was struck-down in the prime of his life with this disease and forced to deal with the many "not-so-great" things that MS offered. And like me, I see how MS has changed his outlook on life, mainly allowing him to develop a more-or-less carefree attitude. When you have a progressive disease like MS you quickly realize that there are many smaller things in life that happen almost daily that don't really matter as much as they once did (i.e. like the motorist who cuts you off on the highway, or the person leaving the store seeing that you are carrying bags in both hands but does not have the courtesy to hold the door open for you, or the inso-lent customer service representative you are speaking with on the tele-phone trying to resolve an issue, or the rude driver who deviously pulls into and "steals" the parking spot you were waiting patiently for at the mall parking lot, or the kid's propensity to leave their dirty dishes and utensils unwashed and in the sink, or the lights they would leave on when leaving their rooms, etc.). When Peter and I talk now, we laugh when we look back on things like that and cannot believe how "pissed off," excited and visibly upset we used to get. Several years after being diagnosed with MS, Peter and I both independently realized that little stuff like this doesn't matter and is not worth getting upset about. In the grand scheme of things, the "little" stuff doesn't matter. Others around us, in particular our spouses, do not get this and frequently consider our nonchalant, carefree attitudes as being insensitive to the events that are happening around us each day. It is only once you have something like MS that you see how small and trivial such things are, and that they are not worth fretting about.

To this day, Peter and I meet for lunch or breakfast about once per month to "shoot the breeze" and catch up on things. We both refuse to let these meetings become gripe sessions. We instead use them to talk about life in general. Initially though we spend the first few minutes or so insulting and poking fun at one another, in a "good-natured" way of course. We then get more serious and take the opportunity to share some things that may be helpful to one another in our daily lives when dealing with MS (i.e. like the time I introduced Peter to a tripod attachment he could purchase to snap on to the bottom of his cane to provide him with greater stability when walking, or the time Peter made me realize that using a motorized scooter or transport chair or a walker was not something to be embarrassed by or ashamed of, or the time that I turned Peter on to visiting the gym and having him make an appointment to see my personal trainer Chris, etc.). Yeah, there are times that Peter and I do complain about things, including the many frustrations we encounter on a daily basis due to our having MS. But these discussions never really go on too far and become gripe sessions, as one of us often lifts the other person up and puts off a soon to become "funk" by making a joke or saying something positive and uplifting. The good thing however is that we share something in common that we can easily relate to and identify with. Then, we temporarily go back to insulting one-another; this certainly helps to lighten the mood! I enjoy these get-togethers with Peter, and always look forward to them!

Generally monthly, if not more frequently, the information sessions hosted by the pharmaceutical companies manufacturing the drugs (i.e. like Avonex, Betaseron, Copaxone, etc.) cover topics relating to relapsing-remitting MS. Since no formal drugs had yet been fully developed and approved by the FDA through 2015 for the secondary progressive and primary progressive forms of the disease, the pharmaceutical companies do not hold information sessions that cover these topics. In addition, there currently is at least one, sometimes two information sessions held per month that are sponsored by Acorda Therapeutics – the makers of Ampyra (aka the MS "walking drug"). These events are always very well attended (no doubt the fact they generally serve fine dinners and lunches helps), with a large number of MS patients attending serving as spokespeople and advocates for the drug (I often wonder if many of them are "plants" from Acorda). The majority of the other people attending these sessions are probably not yet using the drug and likely come with the objective of learning if Ampyra can be helpful and useful for them. I must say that the two or three Ampyra sessions that I have attended, in addition to the food being very good, were all done very well. These sessions provided the audience with some very compelling and convincing information about the drug that likely encouraged and prompted many to speak with their neurologists afterwards about seeing if Ampyra was right for them. Acordia representatives who spoke were always upfront and honest in saying that Amprya did not always work for everyone. They did go on to say, however that because everyone is different, Ampyra is a drug certainly worth considering, particularly in light of the fact that side-effects of the drug (if taken as prescribed) are minimal. To that end, there were always several people scattered throughout the audience that were taking the drug and swore that it made a stark and remarkable difference by improving their gait and walking speed. Unfortunately for me, Ampyra only offered only a very slight benefit and did *not* provide for me the "stark/remarkable" improvements that some MS patients claimed they had experienced. For those people contemplating giving the drug a try, comments made by the drug company and the patient advocates were well received, and I'm sure offered encouragement and hope for many. For me, since I was already taking Ampyra and was familiar with its benefits and effects, the real value for me attending these sessions came from the fact that I was able to meet with and talk with many new people, thus enabling me to gain fresh ideas and perspectives about MS and learn how others were coping. Plus, it was a great way to get a "free" meal!

In addition to the many monthly information sessions put-on by the pharmaceutical companies and their network affiliates, the LI Chapter of the MS Society, the Multiple Sclerosis Association of America (MSAA) and the National Multiple Sclerosis Society (NMSS), the North American Research Committee of Multiple Sclerosis (NARCOMS) also organizes one or two sessions each per year focusing on emerging research and updates on clinical trials. In particular, the MSAA holds an annual half-day session (usually in the fall, in Manhattan and Westchester County) focused solely on MS research trends and current developments. This annual MSAA session, usually sponsored by the Mt. Sinai Medical Center in New York, is always very well attended and consistently features key speakers who are prominent neurologists and researchers in the field. These speakers are usually affiliated with a number of prestigious institutions like Mt. Sinai, the Cleveland Mayo Clinic or the MS Comprehensive Care Center at the University of Southern California (USC), etc. The nice thing about these events is that they are pretty informal. After the presentations conclude and the formal Question and Answer (Q&A) sessions end, the keynote speakers often-times mingle informally with audience members and engage in individual discussions with the participants. They field distinct questions and often share patient stories that put a more humanistic face on MS. To me, this is extremely valuable and gives me an opportunity to talk "one on one" with some of the leading researchers in the MS field, gather business cards, build my network and provide me with a "license" to pick up the telephone and call them down the road to ask questions.

My biggest and only gripe about many of the sessions is that the lunches or dinners offered are presented in a buffet style. Inevitably, I along with many others in attendance, have to rely on someone else to help get the food. Now really, does it make sense to host a session about MS and attended by many MS patients themselves in a restaurant or conference center serving food in a buffet forum? I don't think so!

I always make it a point to attend as many of these sessions as I can and learn as much as possible about MS. Not only is this an invaluable networking opportunity and learning experience, it also gives me ammunition to talk intelligently to my neurologist and ask relevant questions each time I have a scheduled appointment. It also helps me better understand what my neurologist is telling me. Attending these sessions continues to give me the opportunity meet many people for the first time, rekindle some prior friendships and just listen and learn about new things. Plus, it gets me out of the house! Keeping abreast of the latest news about MS is always intriguing and very interesting, to say the least. It's quite amazing how far things have come in the ten years or so since I was first diagnosed. When I received my diagnosis in 2006, there were essentially three drugs on the market that were approved by the FDA (commonly referred to as the "ABC" drugs, i.e. Avonex, Betaseron and Copaxone). All of these drugs required self-injection (either daily, every other day or weekly). Nearly ten years later in 2015, close to one dozen drugs (versus three) are now available and on the market to treat the disease. And several of these treatments are now available in pill form, with a few others administered intravenously (either monthly or more infrequently). While all the MS drugs that have come to market in the ten years since my diagnosis have focused exclusively on treating the relapsing remitting form of the disease, there are several new drugs that are in various clinical trial phases focused on the primary progressive and secondary progressive forms of the disease. In addition, one or two drugs now being tested focus entirely on functionality restoration. This is *very* exciting news! As researchers have made such tremendous progress in ten short years, I can only imagine what things will be like ten years from now when it comes to dealing with, treating and potentially curing MS. Not to come off as being trite, but I cannot help but think about what I often hear so many doctors and researchers say at many of the information sessions and MS gatherings that I often attend, "If you are going to be diagnosed with MS, now is the time!"

Chapter 15

Knowledge is Power: Coming to Grips with Reality

"I n a time of turbulence and change, it is truer than ever that knowledge is power"— *John F. Kennedy*.

These words spoken by John F. Kennedy, the 35th President of the United States, are so very true. When you step back and think, having MS creates tremendous uncertainty due to its ever changing, very turbulent and highly un-predictable nature. This being the case, the more knowledge you have about the disease the better equipped you will likely be to deal with the daily ups and downs that are associated with it and the better equipped you will be in making informed decisions about your various treatment options. You can never have enough knowledge. However, the manner in which one chooses to use the information and knowledge obtained can create issues. Having too much information can result in an unclear and scattered thought process. This may cause one to make hasty decisions and reach pre-mature or inappropriate conclusions. But as John F. Kennedy so concisely implies, it is critical that one amass the knowledge necessary to deal with turbulent and changing situations; possessing knowledge is a pre-condition to having power. It is critical that one draw from a wide range of information sources, discern "the good data from the bad" and consider all the facts available when reaching a final conclusion. Having the right degree of knowledge provides one with the power necessary to make proper and objective decisions, and invoke necessary change.

Ever since being diagnosed with MS in 2006, I always made it a point to do research and learn as much as possible about the disease. As time has moved forward, perhaps the most dangerous and unwieldy source of information I would come across would be from the internet. At first, searching the web gave me a quick and easy way of learning about MS—what it means, the various forms of the disease, the different treatment options available, etc. In a general sense, the web proved to be an excellent information source early on that gave me a broad-spectrum of knowledge about MS. Not even knowing at first what MS was, let alone what it actually stood for, the internet helped me gain familiarity and a basic understanding of the disease. At that point, the information I gleamed from the internet was not dangerous at all. It gave me the basics necessary to begin understanding more about what MS was. The internet became my "MS 101" teaching tool. This was a far cry from grasping and understanding how to use the Dewey Decimal system (for those who may not be familiar with this, I suggest doing a Google search about it). I'm sure you will be astounded to find out how cumbersome it was just a few decades ago to do research and obtain information, and the task required to navigate through card catalogues in public libraries to acquire data.

Early on after my diagnosis, I learned four very basic things that have kept me grounded and have proven essential in broadening my knowledge base about MS. These include:

- Becoming Educated: The more I learned about MS, the less uncertain and fearful I became of what the future would hold and what would happen next. Understanding the disease allowed me to be better prepared to understand it and address some of the challenges that lied ahead. Later on, I learned that education was not only about reading and doing research on the internet but was also very much about acquiring knowledge from others by meeting people, attending information sessions, going to re-search seminars, becoming part of support groups and attending therapy sessions. These actions continually force me today to ask questions and learn more about what I do not know, and also provide me with a core group of people to turn to when I face a challenge and need advice relating to dealing with my condition. I continue to educate myself on new and pertinent information about MS, and acquire a great deal of knowledge and gain tremendous insights by talking with others.

- <u>Writing Things Down:</u> Early on I would keep a journal as a good way of clearing my head, organizing my thoughts and managing my anxiety. Initially this also served as a good tool to use when seeing my neurologist so that I was better prepared and equipped to talk about my symptoms (or initially, the lack thereof). Keeping a journal also helped me early-on to identify sources of stress, isolate critical trigger situations and figure out ways to avoid them. Committing things to paper also helped me organize my thoughts and allowed me to remember impor-tant follow-up items and key questions to ask my doctor. I no longer keep a formal daily journal of events today, and I stopped doing so around 2010. Since being diagnosed in 2006, I have adopted a number of routines to help me get through each day's activities. Therefore, I no longer see the benefits associated with keeping a formal daily journal. After a while, you learn to live with the disease and modify your daily routines and behaviors accordingly without having to rely on a diary or a log to record your feelings, thoughts and activities. At least I have.

- <u>Getting Physical and Exercising:</u> Exercise releases endorphins, the "happiness" hormones known to relieve stress. I was (and still am) very adamant about exercising and remaining active. I read early on, before even starting medical treatments and taking any drugs for my MS, that exercise was frowned upon for those diagnosed with the disease. Today, this is somewhat hard to believe and that thinking has since changed over the past thirty years. Researchers and leading neurologists now strongly recommend that MS patients exercise regularly and remain active. "Keep moving" is the dictum of doctors, caretakers and physical therapists to MS patients today. From my perspective, while it may not always be easy for me on some days to "get out there" and go to the gym or the trainer, doing so helps me to feel better, especially several hours after returning home. In addition, while hard to explain, exercising and remaining active helps me build greater confidence when I am "out and about" meeting with and asking questions of others in order to satisfy my general thirst for knowledge. Aside from the physical benefits associated with exercising and remaining active, doing so also provides me with a mental benefit. Like I say, this is hard to define and explain, but it helps me to build and maintain a high level of self-esteem. My commitment to exercising and staying active on a daily basis is stronger today than ever before. I cannot stress enough its importance. Yes, it has become a bit more difficult today for me to "get out there" and exercise/keep active, but I know it is something I must do!

- <u>Setting Limits on Worrying and Complaining:</u> The NMSS actually recommends devoting up to up to five minutes of each morning and evening to "wallowing." I must admit that wallowing is *not* something that I need to schedule. As time went on after being diagnosed, I quickly came to grips with the fact that it was true—I *did* have MS, and whining and complaining was *not* about to change anything. The only thing that bitching and complaining serves the purpose of doing is to turn "off" others around you instead of bringing them closer to you for strength and support. Instead of whining, I began to channel my energies into more productive ways of figuring out how to modify my daily routines in order to devise workarounds that would allow me to function more normally. Today, the only time that I voice my frustrations and anger is when I'm alone. At times I let out loud yells. These events and displays of emotion are totally unplanned. After a few short minutes of yelling, cursing (I'm actually surprised by some of the foul words I spew out) and screaming, I quickly come back to reality and take a deep breath and think, "Why *not* me?" I truly consider myself fortunate in that in the grand scheme of things, I realize that matters could be much worse. Having MS is not something I would wish on anyone, but I realize now that there are much worse things in life that I could be dealing with. And at least for the time being, MS is here to stay and is something that I must continue to deal with.

As time marched on and 2006 turned into 2007, I sought out information about MS by relying exclusively on the internet and reading as much as I could about the disease (in brochures, flyers, email notifications, etc.). I firmly believed that the more I knew about MS and the better educated I became, the easier it would be for me to make more informed treatment decisions. The only problem: My source of information and knowledge was mostly isolated and "one-sided," as the vast majority of it came from the internet.

What wound up happening was that I became inundated with information and started looking into alternative therapies that were in addition to the medications I was taking. This is not necessarily a bad thing, if approached in a thoughtful and orderly manner. I remember trying some pretty wacky alternative treatments, which I discuss in an earlier chapter. There was little doubt that I had become "data rich and information poor," and started believing what I wanted to believe. I later realized that for every topic I'd read about on the internet there were numerous pro and con positions that were espoused. If I wanted something to be true I would search the web until I found articles, statements and statistics that supported my hypothesis. I focused exclusively on finding data that would defend and support my beliefs, rather than obtaining information objectively from a variety of sources that would provide me with a more balanced set of facts that I could use as a basis for making decisions and reaching conclusions. On several occasions right after being diagnosed when I went into see my neurologist, I would bring up a subject and make a statement regarding something that I had just read about on the internet (either a clinical trial that was recently launched, or a new drug pending approval by the FDA, etc.), and say something like ... "I was looking on the internet and read about this clinical trial underway, or learned about research and testing being done about [xyz] drug that in early testing showed some positive effects on reducing or eliminating MS symptoms in laboratory mice." The first few times that I brought something like this up in a discussion with Dr. Blitz, I remember her telling me, "You're not a mouse" and that I should "stop believing everything [you read] on the internet." After about the second or third time I went to see and greeted Dr. Blitz in this manner, I stopped making such inquiries and statements and instead replaced them with a simple question I would ask at each appointment, and still ask to this day: "Any cure yet?"

I begin every appointment I have with Dr. Blitz asking this question, and am hopeful that one of these days she will pleasantly surprise me and respond to my "any cure yet" question with something like … *"funny you should ask—a new drug has been approved by the FDA which restores functionality …."* The reality of the situation however was that for the first few years after my diagnosis I continued scouring the web for as much data and information that I could find about the disease. I just became a little more cautious about becoming over-zealous and bringing to Dr. Blitz's attention every little factoid that I uncovered. After all, she is the doctor, *not me!* And when a treatment becomes available that undoes some of the damage caused by MS, I am certain she will enthusiastically let me know.

By 2007, use of the internet for conducting research throughout the world became quite pervasive. In addition, thousands of health-oriented websites, medical blogs and even doctor-based television and radio programs were emerging. The good news here was that I had more opportunities than ever to take charge of my own medical care. However, the daily bombardment of news reports and drug advertisements provided me with little guidance on how to make sense of all the self-proclaimed medical breakthroughs, claims for a cure and worrisome risks. My challenge: To decode the latest health news about MS so I could gain the knowledge necessary to talk intelligently with Dr. Blitz in order to play a more active role in my own medical care. I had to balance this with the fact that as I said before, Dr. Blitz and not me was the doctor and as such I had to remain conscious and fully aware about any "new" information I would consider. I believed that the more knowledge I possessed about MS, the more in control I would be of my situation. In reality, I later learned that this was not necessarily the case.

It wasn't about having more information but rather about having the right information. Information overload is something to be aware of and there is certainly a fine balance between empowering yourself with the right level of knowledge and amassing too much information. For some people, more information makes them totally overwrought and obsessed, while others get more relaxed, feel more confident, become more comfortable and become further empowered. So for the three years or so after my diagnosis, I became an "MS information junkie" and secretly hoped that I would uncover some breakthrough medical study or a cure buried somewhere on the internet. Instead, I became fully aware of a series of stem cell clinical trials being performed in places like Mexico, Costa Rica, Argentina, Europe, etc., and frequently came across some very frightening statistics about MS.

While statistics provided me with some valuable information, they often led to my becoming obsessed with the disease instead of letting go and moving on. While they did offer me a better understanding of some of the risks associated with the disease and some of the various treatment options available, I was careful not to have them become a deciding factor in determining my care. This was a fine balancing act—one that I admittedly still struggle with today. It is so exciting to read about some miracle treatment or therapy for MS that has emerged that you become temporarily blinded from reality and are tempted to make a rash decision to try it. I am now wise enough to stop and think about what Dr. Blitz would always tell me—that I should stop believing everything that is posted on the internet. As time continues to move forward I have gained a much better understanding of why she says this. The reality is that when a miracle therapy or drug is discovered, it will certainly be top level headline news that will be carried across all major television, radio, print and social media outlets. Everyone will be talking about it and rest assured it will not be something buried on page three of some google internet search.

By around 2010 or so I began to realize that searching the web to acquire knowledge about MS was not the greatest use of my time nor was it the "be-all and end-all." Much of the information I got from the internet was either exaggerated, plain false or just right-out scary! I learned there is a lot more to decoding one's health than by placing reliance solely on information obtained from the web. It was critical to speak openly with your doctor, your family and other MS patients. It was also critical to attend information sessions to meet people and participate in support groups. These are additional things that hold tremendous value. Moreover, books and magazines are also a very beneficial source of information. The internet represents only one tool available to garner information and like anything else, putting all your eggs in one basket is not a wise thing to do. Like any good investment advisor will tell you, diversify! Doing medical research and investing your money is no different in this regard, and diversification is critical!

In particular though, I discovered that attending information sessions and participating in support groups was a great way to learn more about the disease and get a better feel for how others were coping and dealing with it. Additionally, I began attending annual and semi-annual research sessions where tons of information would be presented. I would then use the internet to conduct additional research to supplement the information that I had already become aware of. One thing I realized was that the MS landscape was rapidly changing and that new information was becoming available almost weekly. Numerous clinical trials started surfacing regularly. It seems like since 2013, another new drug for treating relapsing remitting MS was coming to market almost quarterly. The information and knowledge that I was acquiring was now becoming more precise, and unlike the randomness associated with my prior web-based searches, the knowledge I was acquiring was becoming much more focused, objective and balanced.

One piece of information that I found most intriguing discussed Mitochondria, often referred to as the powerhouse of the cell. Mitochondria generate the energy that cells needed to do their jobs. For example, brain cells need a lot of energy to be able to communicate with each other and also to communicate with parts of the body that may be very far away from the "command center," or the brain. As such, messages need to be transported along the cells and need lots of energy. Muscle fibers also need a lot of energy to promote movement, maintain posture and assist with the lifting of objects. Mitochondria generate chemical energy (similar to the type of energy that is released from a battery) that is called adenosine triphosphate (or ATP for short). ATP is an energy currency that every cell in the body uses and helps support life. The machinery that the mitochondria use to make ATP is called the electron transport chain, which is made up of several protein groups that work together to carry out their function. The whole theory behind there being a "cell powerhouse" makes perfect sense to me, and a number of dietary routines have begun to emerge that support enhanced and more precise targeting of mitochondria care. To date, I have only lightly touched on some of these dietary routines (i.e. like doing my best to increase my intake of fruits and vegetables each day, reducing the amount of processed foods consumed, improving the overall quality and freshness of foods consumed daily, drinking green juice derived from blended fruits and vegetables, drinking plenty of water, reducing my sugar intake, etc.). To date I have not yet adopted any specific diet to help with my MS. I guess time will only tell where I go from here. A vitamin supplement called Mito-Q has also emerged which supposedly protects mitochondria and helps the body to produce more energy and reduce fatigue. We'll see....

As John F. Kennedy reminds us, "In times of turbulence and change, it is truer than ever that knowledge is power." In a nutshell, here are some of the key pieces of knowledge that I have acquired and revelations that I have made about MS since I was diagnosed in 2006. These facts, feelings and thoughts have given me the wisdom and power necessary to move forward and help me balance (no pun intended) the *reality* that *I do have* the disease, together with the reality that drives me to *live life to its fullest* each and every day. I continue coming to grips with the reality that for now, I have MS and as such have to figure out the best way to remain as active and as fully integrated into society as I possibly can.

The following offers a simple snapshot of some of the basic things I have come to realize since being diagnosed with MS. It is a work in progress, as I'm sure if I were to compose a similar catalog two years or so down the road after publishing this book, I would most likely have a number of additions, changes and deletions.

In the meantime, here goes:

MS Is Unpredictable
- No two people with MS progress in the same manner—it's not one size fits all;
- MS symptoms can change on a weekly, daily or sometimes hourly basis;
- MS can literally and figuratively knock you off your feet at any time;
- MS is like an assorted box of chocolates, in that you never know what's inside until you get it;
- MS is like a roller coaster...you have ups and downs, twists and turns: The exception being that unlike a roller coaster, MS is never fun;
- MS robs you of your self-worth every day by stealing the little things you may have been able to do the day before;
- Heat and humidity are not friends of MS; and

- Just because yesterday was a bad day doesn't mean today will be.

MS Is Real: It's Not an Excuse

- I'm not faking it and I'm not being a hypochondriac or lazy, I just feel "off" at times and need to rest;
- Not being able to do the simple things in life (like walking well, puttering around the house, impulsively going to a store or a shopping mall, etc.) is very frustrating;
- MS is exhausting, and often times causes extreme fatigue;
- MS is *not* something one chooses, and is out of a person's control; however, figuring out various workarounds to make daily living a bit less challenging *is* within one's control; and
- Remain determined, stay optimistic and don't give up!

MS Is Not a Death Sentence (and Is Not Contagious)!

- While having MS is a struggle one must deal with daily, it is a struggle that can make a person stronger;
- MS is not fatal, and isn't always debilitating;
- MS doesn't change who you are, just what you can do;
- MS is a terribly frightening diagnosis to receive: But with time and education, it's not the end of the world, and there are worse things in life to deal with;
- It is very simple to become obsessed with information about MS. The key is to get the proper and right amount of information, use it wisely and not let it drive everything you do; and
- Having the right amount of information and knowledge can be very helpful, but having too much information can lead to arriving at inappropriate conclusions and making hasty decisions; this is not a good thing!

MS Is Oftentimes Stressful and Depressing

- MS slowly and quietly takes away one's mobility, and may over time lessen one's cognitive thinking abilities;
- MS can very quickly rob a person of their dignity and self-esteem;
- MS is not at all easy to live with—physically, mentally and emotionally;
- Meeting with and talking to others who have MS is priceless, as it provides a strong support base that is helpful in gaining insights about how others are dealing with daily challenges and coping emotionally; and
- The more people [with MS] that one meet's and talks to, the more a person realizes and learns that nearly everybody has their own cross to bear (whether it be a medical issue, a family problem, a financial issue, etc.).

MS Is a Constant Battle, For Everyone

- MS is devastating—not just to the person having the disease, but also to the entire family. Never forget that MS has a marked impact on a person's loved ones and "caretaker(s)";
- MS requires those who love us to be open minded, be 'warm' and have great big hearts;
- MS is something that patients have on their minds daily, even on days when they are feeling fine; however, most people cannot help but think about what the future will hold, as this is only natural; and
- It is critical for those supporting MS patients (i.e. caretakers, loved ones, etc.) to *not* take away their independence, but instead balance daily support needs without stripping a person of their dignity and self-esteem.

Exercise and Remain Active

- Exercising and remaining physically active provides enormous benefits to both physical and mental wellbeing;
- You pay to change the oil in your car and rotate the tires, so why not pay to maintain your own body by joining a gym or purchasing an exercise bike?; and
- It is critical to remain active and engaged in the workforce (if possible), as this is an essential factor for overall wellbeing; doing so helps keep a person abreast of current marketplace events, allows one to maintain relationships, fosters networking with others and provides a strong sense of confidence and accomplishment.

MS Still Has No Cure

- MS can't be fixed quickly with any miracle potion that may be publicized;
- Do not rush to seek out sensationalized stem cell and other alternative therapies touted outside the country;
- More MS research is needed for a treatment and a cure; and
- Don't believe everything you read on the internet!

Don't Sweat the Little Things

- Put things into perspective, as the small stuff is not worth fretting over;
- Learn to differentiate and deal with relevant issues versus those that are inconsequential; and
- Remember that there are bigger things in life that many people around you are dealing with daily.

Stop Whining!

- Sulking, moaning, complaining and whining will not bring about a cure for MS any faster, and it only chases people away. Instead, keep a positive attitude, stay optimistic and remain up-beat;
- Complaining brings down others, so don't do it;
- It is an understatement when you tell others around you who do not suffer with MS that "they have no idea what it is like having MS"; voicing this truthful fact accomplishes nothing except to make others feel bad, so don't say it; and
- Step back, reflect and realize you are not immortal and ask yourself, "Why *not* me?"

It is indeed unfortunate to have been diagnosed with this disease. However, having MS has really helped me come to grips with reality, prioritize critical things and make me realize what is truly important in life. The little annoyances in life really do not matter as much to me, so getting "worked up" about them rarely happens to me anymore. If having this disease has taught me anything it has given me the knowledge and resultant power necessary to navigate the turbulent, ever changing and highly unpredictable road ahead called the "MS Highway."

Chapter 16

Restoring Functionality and Looking Ahead to the Future

It is interesting as I step back and reflect about how much things have evolved over the last twenty years pertaining to MS research. It is hard to believe that the first therapy approved for the treatment of MS came to market in 1993/1994, with the introduction of interferon beta 1b (Betaseron). At the time of my writing this book (2015), nearly one dozen therapies have been approved by the Federal Drug Administration (FDA) specifically for the treatment of the disease. The good news today is that there are more potential MS therapies in development than in any other time in history. And since I was diagnosed with the disease in 2006, the number of treatment options available has nearly quadrupled. This is exciting and is great news, right? Well, not exactly. For many suffering or newly diagnosed with the disease, this is indeed terrific. However, for those of us who have been battling the disease for a number of years (like myself), while the upsurge in MS research is certainly exciting it is still somewhat frustrating. Why? Because as of 2015, every drug currently available in the market and approved by the FDA is targeted to treat the relapsing remitting form of the disease, with nothing yet on the market to help treat primary progressive or secondary progressive MS. Plus all of the drugs that have been approved to date either slow disease progression, ease symptoms, moderately or temporarily improve function or decrease the frequency and/or severity of relapses. To date though nothing is yet available to stop the disease in its entirety or restore functions that have been lost. At the time when I was diagnosed in 2006, there was little belief that nervous system repair was even possible. Since then, through the tireless efforts of the National MS Society, numerous other funding partners, pharmaceutical companies, doctors and researchers around the world, a whole new field has emerged dedicated to the pursuit of strategies to repair the nervous system and restore function to people with MS. Now *this* is exciting news!

With MS, the immune system attacks the brain and spinal cord causing damage to nerve fibers and their protective myelin coating. Without proper myelin coating, nerve fibers fail to conduct and transmit signals properly which leads to a various array of symptoms which can result in long term disability. In short, the "get moving" signals which are sent from the brain to the muscles aren't reaching their target in a timely way. Restoring what's been lost in MS requires a more thorough understanding of how nerves and myelin work normally and how repair can be stimulated. A great deal of research continues being done to identify agents capable of regenerating myelin. One such study pertains to research being done with mesenchymal stem cells (or MSCs), where an initial clinical trial (Phase I) was successfully completed in 2014/2015 with no significant safety issues noted. A phase II trial is now underway at the Cleveland clinic that is further examining the technique's safety. Additionally, it will focus more directly on patient benefits. Clearly scientists still have a long way to go before a treatment is found that effectively tackles the root causes of MS. Based on the encouraging results seen thus far, other clinical trials are now commencing and beginning to enroll patients. This not only relates to mesenchymal stem cells, but other stem cell approaches as well (i.e. hematopoietic stem cell transplantation, or HSCT, etc.). Essentially, HSCT involves a reset of the immune system where patients are injected with a drug that stimulates stem cells, allowing them to multiply. A filtering process is then undertaken whereby patients are subsequently injected with their own hematopoietic stem cells to virtually erase and re-set the immune system (admittedly though, this sounds very scary). This is done with the hope of abolishing the autoimmunity responsible for MS, the theory being that when the immune system comes back it will cease attacking the brain. In one related research study, MS patients showed improvements in limb strength, walking, movement control and vision for greater than one year after the infusion. While one needs to keep in mind that while these results pertain only to one study, they are nonetheless very encouraging. There is a great deal of optimism today relating to stem cell research and many researchers believe that it may provide a cure for the condition in the near future. Let's all keep our fingers crossed and wait to see what happens!

Perhaps equally or even more encouraging than the work being done with stem cells is work being done by researchers relating to a protein we all have in our bodies, called LINGO-1. Specifically, LINGO-1 is a protein in the central nervous system that regulates myelination. The cells making up all organs in the body receive "instructions" from this protein regarding when to grow and when to cease growing myelin. Without these cellular "checks and balances," tissues could grow without restraint and potentially cause some malignancies. LINGO-1 remains active and at work in our bodies until the human nervous system is fully developed, usually shortly at or shortly after the onset of adolescence. At this point in life, enough myelin has been produced and further production is no longer necessary. By unblocking this protein, a drug called Anti-LINGO-1 is now being studied. Anti-LINGO-1 is an agent with potential remyelinative properties that has shown in several animal studies the ability to promote spinal cord remyelination. Effectively, Anti-LINGO-1 tells the body, "Hey body, the vacation is over. Time to start growing myelin again!" This, in theory may reverse or repair any damage previously caused by MS. The trick will be to regulate this "on-off switch" so that myelin growth is stopped after a certain trigger point is reached and then only restarted, as necessary, if MS choses to attack again. Researchers fear that by growing myelin without restraint and being unable to "flick the switch to off," dangerous malignancies and other side-effects could result. Therefore, this is a critical component of Anti-LINGO-1 research.

Early trials of Anti-LINGO-1 have been conducted thus far for MS patients suffering from optic neuritis. An initial mesenchymal stem cell trial was also done focusing on the optic nerve. The results of these trials are promising and show a number of patients having their nerve signals between the retina and the brain restored to normal or nearly normal. This likely occurred due to re-generation of myelin along the optic nerve, but the exact cause of the beneficial effect has not yet been fully determined. Researchers are now (in 2015) following up with these patients to study the permanency of these results. Anti-LINGO-1 could reverse the damage of Multiple Sclerosis, virtually "curing" balance, vision and other problems for MS sufferers. In addition, researchers thus far have found Anti-LINGO-1 to be generally well tolerated, with the overall incidence and severity of adverse effects being quite minimal. Bottom line: Early results provide an encouraging indication that Anti-LINGO-1 appears safe and may facilitate remyelination! Studies regarding mesenchymal stem cell research are also very encouraging.

Current human trials of Anti-LINGO-1 leverage research which is aimed at stimulating the body's natural healing abilities. Blockading this protein with the monoclonal antibody, Anti-LINGO-1, is indeed cutting edge. A second larger Phase II trial (called SYNERGY) is now underway to look at this drug's effectiveness specifically for individuals having either RRMS or SPMS. While Anti-LINGO-1 is not a cure for MS, it is something that has certainly gotten my attention. "BIG TIME!" This research has truly confirmed my belief that there will soon be a day when those having MS will be able the avail themselves to two treatment options which can be taken simultaneously. The first—being taking one of the existing drugs currently approved by the FDA (i.e. Betaseron, Avonex, Tecfidera, Copaxone, etc.) aimed at slowing MS progression and thereby minimizing or preventing further destruction of myelin. The second - being taking a drug like Anti-LINGO-1 which will help to re-generate myelin that may have already been damaged. So, my theory is that MS will continue to exist until a real "cure" is found. However, MS will no longer be able to wreak the sustained havoc that it does today on many patients due to the combination of two drugs that can be taken together. Hence, lost functionality will be restored and new damage will no longer occur.

In addition to the excitement surrounding stem cell research and the ongoing trials for Anti-LINGO-1, there are some other interesting things I have been reading about when it comes to MS research and what the future holds. Some seem odd and non-conventional, like work being done to develop a nasal vaccine which is intended to enhance the immune system's ability to regulate itself. From here, the antibodies developed and contained in the nasal spray would travel to the immune system where they would forefend any attacks on the central nervous system. Similarly, there is another seemingly non-conventional research study which is focused on developing a skin patch. If research continues and successful trials for these two studies are to hold up, there would no longer be any need for needles or lengthy infusions, just a quick spray into the rich mucosal lining of the nose or a patch affixed to one's skin (similar to the Nicoderm patch used to stop smoking). This is indeed very interesting!

Another study that has perked my interest relates to a drug called Siponimod (or BAF312), which is a cousin to the drug Gilenya that was the first oral disease-modifying MS treatment approved in 2011 by the FDA for RRMS. A Phase III trial of Siponimod was launched in 2013 to specifically focus on SPMS, after findings done in earlier trials indicated that patients treated with the drug had a reduction of nearly 80 percent in active MRI lesions. The goal of the Phase III study is to determine if improvements in disability progression for patients having SPMS, as measured by the EDSS scale, can be achieved. This is important and helps buy time as research continues with some of the other restorative therapies. Compared to Gilenya, Siponimod has a relatively short half-life which means that the drug does not stay in the body as long. Researchers hope this will minimize some of the side-effects, mainly cardiac issues (i.e. lower heart rate) that have occurred since the introduction to the market of Gilenya. It is the cardiac issue that scares me the most, so for that reason I think I'll wait for the Phase III trial results to become final before considering if BAF312 is right for me. Having MS is enough to worry about and deal with. No sense muddying the waters with cardiac issues. Still though, the Siponimod trial is very promising.

Researchers are also actively studying monoclonal antibodies, which are derived from cells that are identical (cloned from a single cell and then replicated). Monoclonal antibodies are key in that they can be specifically targeted to perform a particular action. This is significant when trying to impact a structure as complex as the human immune system. There are some treatments for MS already approved by the FDA that are derived from monoclonal antibodies (i.e. Natalizumab or Tysabri, Alemtuzumab or Lemtrada, etc.). Others are in various stages of research, experimentation and clinical trial. Another study being done relates to Vitamin D levels and the fact that individuals with higher Vitamin D levels showed lower numbers of gadolinium enhancing lesions appearing on MRIs. Many of the clinical trials being done here use Vitamin D as an add-on to existing therapies to see if supplemental amounts of the vitamin have any disease modifying effects. So true to form, I have increased my daily intake of Vitamin D over the last few years by taking a vitamin supplement. As such, I have improved my Vitamin D blood level count by 50 percent (or from thirty to sixty). I do not feel any different as a result. But hey, popping an extra vitamin pill each day can't hurt (I think). Taking one extra pill per day is something I'll have to eventually get used to anyway when the Anti-LINGO-1 treatment hits the market (I assume it will be a pill). If successful, repairing the damaged nervous system will be an enormous paradigm shift in how MS is dealt with, is viewed by patients and is treated by the medical community!

As has been told to me by doctors numerous times, now is a great time to have MS. Still I'm not sure if it is ever a good time to have such a dreadful disease. I guess the point here is that because such great things are happening today in the MS research arena, those afflicted with the condition have more hope than ever before that a "cure" will be discovered. The momentum here is great and is undoubtedly very exciting. In my mind, it's not *if* a cure will be found, but rather it is *when* a cure will be found!

So, I continue to give money on a regular basis to the National MS Society. While my ongoing contributions are probably insignificant in the grand scheme of things, I'm hopeful that others will open their wallets to give generously and help spur the drive to find a cure. I'm sure that more funding can only help the cause. This is why I get so angry when billions of dollars are spent by our government each year and given to countries that burn our flag and hate us. I will never understand why these funds are not being allocated toward medical research focused of finding new drugs and cures for people having chronic medical conditions, like Parkinsoin's Disease, Lupus, Cancer, MS, etc.

Epilogue

As I close in on ten years since being diagnosed with MS in 2006, I can honestly say it has been an interesting (and very frustrating) ride, at that. I have gone from feeling great every day and having no visible symptoms at all, to feeling tired at the end of most days, to walking with a cane and having to navigate balance issues almost daily. In the overall scheme of things though, I guess I'm pretty lucky, as I am still doing "okay."

I must admit for the first few years after being diagnosed I was in denial that I even had MS, especially since I was feeling fine, was able to walk freely and maintain normal balance. My leg strength was great and I had no visible MS symptoms. I felt I could do anything that I once did, and even if I could not, I would never admit it. Still today, on rare occasions I think that I can do almost anything and go anywhere. But within a few short minutes after attempting to do certain tasks, I quickly come back down to earth and face the reality that I just cannot do it. Yes, I have MS. And I need to be realistic about what I can *and* cannot do.

As time has gone on, I have become reliant on a cane to help me walk and keep from losing my balance. I have even broke down and recently purchased a very light three wheel aluminum rollator/walker that

307

I have started using when commuting into New York City. I have become more intolerant of the heat and humidity during the summertime, and am unable to do many of the simple daily things that I once did (i.e. like washing the car or cleaning out the garage, etc.). I am fatigued at the end of most days and now experience intermittent bladder urgency and voiding issues. I have gradually begun to realize that my disease is progressing, albeit slowly. In addition, while I have continued going to the gym and seeing my personal trainer a few times each week, I have cut back and no longer workout five/six days per week like I once did. (That's okay since some of my shirts were getting a bit tight anyway). Going there is just too much of a hassle, so I do whatever exercises I can do at home to stay active and limber. I still leave the house and go to the gym and see my trainer an average of three times per week though! I find pushing myself to "get out there" gives me the confidence necessary to live a relatively "normal" lifestyle.

Today, I remain as active as I can and stay as positive as possible. I know that research will eventually prove successful and that a therapy or a "cure" will be found to restore function lost to this horrible monster called MS. I will not give up! I commute into New York City for work most days of the week, travel out of state to visit clients on rare occasions when necessary and attend client lunches or dinners at times. And yes, I continue to drive! On several occasions since being diagnosed, I have switched and tried different FDA approved medications and have availed myself to various alternative therapies. Call me naïve, but I'm convinced I will come across something one day that will make a noticeable difference. When I think about all that's happened since the first drug approved to treat MS came on the scene in the early 1990s (Betaseron), plus all the progress made in just the last few years to find new treatments to control the disease and along with the aggressive pursuit of strategies to repair the nervous system and restore function to people with MS, I am amazed. Granted, the "cure" cannot come fast enough. But rest assured though, it will come. In the meantime, I just have to stay in good physical shape, keep moving, maintain a positive attitude, steer away from letting depression take over and resist the temptation to say things like, "Why me?" As many will remind me, I just have to "keep smyelin'!"

Comparatively speaking, I guess I'm not in such a bad place after all and things could be a lot worse. So, I continue to plod along, remain thankful that I'm able to do what I can do, stand with my head held high and shout out (or at least think about shouting out), "Why *not* me?"

I'm confident that sometime in the near future, MS will no longer stand for Multiple Sclerosis, but rather stand for "*Mystery Solved*"!

For all those in my life that continue to support me, thank you again...and please, *be patient*! I know that my feelings of anger and frustration come through from time to time, as much as I try to mask them. I try not to be a burden on others, and will do whatever I can (by myself) for as long as I can. Remaining as independent as I can be is very important to me. So please, work with me. Today, MS is real and is something that I must deal with. I am determined to persevere. I continue to adapt and modify my daily routines to the greatest extent possible, and will not give-up. Hopefully, it will not be all that much longer until I can speak in the past tense about a disease I once had...a disease called Multiple Sclerosis!

MS...*Mystery Solved*—let's hope!

About the Author

V incent Spoto was born in Queens, New York (NY) in March, 1959. He is the son of Joseph and Rosalie Spoto (both deceased), and the youngest of three brothers. Vincent was raised in Richmond Hill, Queens NY where he lived in the same house for twenty-five years, until he moved-out when he was married in 1984. For nearly thirty years, Vincent enjoyed a successful career in both Commercial and Investment Banking. In 2007, Vincent launched a very successful consulting and advisory business (RRMS Advisors), which he operates today as one of three founding partners.

In August 2006, Vincent was diagnosed with Multiple Sclerosis (MS) after experiencing intermittent instances of fatigue, an occasional stumble and noticing heaviness in both legs when doing some routine yard work. For nearly one year before he was formally diagnosed, doctors were not certain what, if anything, was wrong and initially suspected Lyme disease. After seeing three separate neurologists and undergoing a series of examinations and tests - including a number of Evoked Potential Tests (EPTs), several Magnetic Resonance Imaging (MRI) tests and a lumbar puncture (spinal tap) - Lyme disease was ruled out and a conclusive diagnosis of MS was made.

Throughout the first few years that followed, Vincent's symptoms were virtually invisible. It wasn't until 2010 when his symptoms slowly became more apparent and he began utilizing a cane to help walk. Thereafter, he began to open-up and tell others about his condition.

Today, Vincent remains fully ambulatory. His MS however, has slowly progressed and has created many challenges for him when performing day-to-day activities.

Together with his wife Luisa and their two daughters (Deanna and Lauren), Vincent continues to remain active and persevere. He remains confident that researchers will discover a cure in his lifetime. In the interim, he is committed to remaining fit, and has devised a number of shortcuts and workarounds to maintain a high degree of independence when performing daily tasks. Vincent remains dedicated to helping others, and decided to write this book in order to share his story and inspire other MS sufferers with a number of 'feel-good' routines that he has adopted in order to live life to the fullest. He also encourages others to see a doctor and get 'checked-out' when they are just not feeling right, and not to simply dismiss certain things (like fatigue, balance issues, heaviness in the limbs, etc.) and attribute them to "just getting old."

"Why _Not_ Me?" provides an insightful look into Vincent's life with MS. It reinforces the theme that remaining active and keeping a positive attitude is critical, and that there are worse things in life to be burdened with besides having MS.

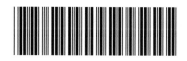

CPSIA information can be obtained
at www.ICGtesting.com
Printed in the USA
LVHW010412160720
660525LV00004B/143